Working with Families of Young Children with Special Needs

WHAT WORKS FOR SPECIAL-NEEDS LEARNERS

Karen R. Harris and Steve Graham
Editors

Strategy Instruction for Students with Learning Disabilities
Robert Reid and Torri Ortiz Lienemann

Teaching Mathematics to Middle School Students with Learning Difficulties
Marjorie Montague and Asha K. Jitendra, Editors

Teaching Word Recognition:
Effective Strategies for Students with Learning Difficulties
Rollanda E. O'Connor

Teaching Reading Comprehension to Students with Learning Difficulties
Janette K. Klingner, Sharon Vaughn, and Alison Boardman

Promoting Self-Determination in Students with Developmental Disabilities
*Michael L. Wehmeyer with Martin Agran, Carolyn Hughes, James E. Martin,
Dennis E. Mithaug, and Susan B. Palmer*

Instructional Practices for Students with Behavioral Disorders:
Strategies for Reading, Writing, and Math
J. Ron Nelson, Gregory J. Benner, and Paul Mooney

Working with Families of Young Children with Special Needs
R. A. McWilliam, Editor

Promoting Executive Function in the Classroom
Lynn Meltzer

Working with Families of Young Children with Special Needs

edited by

R. A. McWilliam

Series Editors' Note by Karen R. Harris and Steve Graham

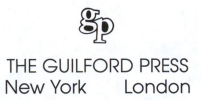

THE GUILFORD PRESS
New York   London

© 2010 The Guilford Press
A Division of Guilford Publications, Inc.
72 Spring Street, New York, NY 10012
www.guilford.com

Printed in the United States of America

This book is printed on acid-free paper.

Last digit is print number: 9 8 7 6 5 4 3 2 1

Library of Congress Cataloging-in-Publication Data

Working with families of young children with special needs / edited by R.A. McWilliam.
    p. cm. — (What works for special-needs learners)
  Includes bibliographical references and index.
  ISBN 978-1-60623-539-3 (pbk.: alk. paper)
  1. Children with disabilities—Education (Early childhood)   2. Early childhood special
education.   3. Early childhood education—Parent participation.   I. McWilliam, R. A.
  LC4019.3.W67 2010
  371.9′0472—dc22

                                                          2009046577

About the Editor

R. A. McWilliam, PhD, is Director of the Center for Child and Family Research at Siskin Children's Institute, a pioneering and far-reaching nonprofit organization for children, families, and professionals in Chattanooga, and Professor in the College of Health, Education and Professional Studies at the University of Tennessee at Chattanooga. He develops interventions for young children with disabilities that always involve the children's families; conducts research on the development of individualized family service plans, child engagement, and service delivery methods; and provides consultation, training, and technical assistance throughout the United States. Dr. McWilliam has served as Director of the Center for Child Development at Vanderbilt University Medical Center and as Senior Scientist at the Frank Porter Graham Child Development Institute at the University of North Carolina at Chapel Hill. He is past president of the Division for Research of the Council for Exceptional Children and past editor of the *Journal of Early Intervention*. Dr. McWilliam is the author of *Family-Centered Intervention Planning: A Routines-Based Resource* (1992) and of the upcoming *Routines-Based Early Intervention* (in press); the editor of *Rethinking Pull-Out Services in Early Intervention: A Professional Resource* (1996); and the coauthor, with Amy M. Casey, of *Engagement of Every Child in the Preschool Classroom* (2007).

Contributors

Mary Beth Bruder, PhD, Departments of Pediatrics and Educational Psychology, and A. J. Pappanikou Center for Excellence in Developmental Disabilities Education, Research, and Service, University of Connecticut, Farmington, Connecticut

Carl J. Dunst, PhD, Orelena Hawks Puckett Institute, Asheville, North Carolina

Lise Fox, PhD, Florida Center for Inclusive Communities, College of Behavioral and Community Sciences, University of South Florida, Tampa, Florida

Marci J. Hanson, PhD, Department of Special Education, San Francisco State University, San Francisco, California

Lee Ann Jung, PhD, Special Education and Rehabilitation Counseling, University of Kentucky, Lexington, Kentucky

Eleanor W. Lynch, PhD, Department of Special Education, San Diego State University, San Diego, California

P. J. McWilliam, PhD, Department of Special Education, Vanderbilt University, Nashville, Tennessee

R. A. McWilliam, PhD, Center for Child and Family Research, Siskin Children's Institute, and College of Health, Education and Professional Studies, University of Tennessee at Chattanooga, Chattanooga, Tennessee

Melinda Raab, PhD, Orelena Hawks Puckett Institute, Asheville, North Carolina

Dathan D. Rush, EdD, CCC-SLP, Family, Infant and Preschool Program, J. Iverson Riddle Developmental Center, Morganton, North Carolina

M'Lisa L. Shelden, PT, PhD, Family, Infant and Preschool Program, J. Iverson Riddle Developmental Center, Morganton, North Carolina

Jennifer Swanson, PhD, Heartland Area Education Agency, Johnston, Iowa

Carol M. Trivette, PhD, Orelena Hawks Puckett Institute, Asheville, North Carolina

Series Editors' Note

When Dr. Smith dies, he goes directly to the pearly gates, where he sees a large group of people waiting to get into heaven. Ignoring the crowd, Dr. Smith walks to the front of the line and informs St. Peter that he is a doctor and wants to go through the gate. In no uncertain terms, he is told to go to the end of the line. "But you don't understand," he complains, "I am a doctor!"

A few minutes later, another person goes to the head of the line and tells St. Peter he wants to enter heaven too. St. Peter also tells him to go to the end of the line, and the man exclaims, "You don't understand, I am Dr. Jones!"

As the two doctors stand at the end of the line commiserating, they spot another man approaching St. Peter. This man is wearing a lab coat, with a stethoscope hanging from his neck. After saying something to St. Peter, he enters heaven.

Irritated, the two doctors approach St. Peter and ask why "that man" did not have to stand in line. A man further back in line replies, "Oh, that's just God. He thinks he's a doctor!"

This joke illustrates a simple but powerful truth—sometimes professionals act as if they and their opinions are more important than the clients they serve. In *Working with Families of Young Children with Special Needs*, R. A. McWilliam and his contributors hold a different view about the relationship between professionals and clients, who, in this case, are families of young children with disabilities. The role of professionals in early childhood special education is to support families in a friendly and collaborative manner, while at the same time providing families and other caregivers with supports necessary for their children to learn needed skills within the context of everyday routines.

Just as important, Dr. McWilliam and his contributors emphasize that special education and early childhood professionals need to concentrate on more than just a child's competence. They advocate a balanced approach to working with families, in which quality of life is valued.

You are in for a great ride, as the message in this book is not only family friendly, but extremely practical. It combines a solid foundation of research, along with a good dose of common sense, tempered by considerable experience in working with young children with special needs and their families. Get ready to learn about ecomaps, routine-based interviews, the primary-coach approach, family centeredness, and more.

This book is part of the series What Works for Special-Needs Learners. The series addresses a significant need in the education of learners with special needs—students who are at risk, those with disabilities, and all children and adolescents who struggle with learning or behavior. Researchers in special education, educational psychology, curriculum and instruction, and other fields have made great progress in understanding what works for struggling learners, yet the practical application of this research base remains quite limited. This is due, in part, to the lack of appropriate materials for teachers, teacher educators, and in-service teacher development programs. Books in this series present assessment, instructional, and classroom management methods with a strong research base and provide specific "how-to" instructions and examples of the use of proven procedures in schools. All volumes in the series are thorough and detailed and facilitate the implementation of evidence-based practices in classrooms and schools.

KAREN R. HARRIS
STEVE GRAHAM

Contents

Introduction   1
R. A. MCWILLIAM

Purpose of the Book   *1*
Basic Themes   *4*
Voices in the Chapters   *4*
Early Intervention/Early Childhood Special Education Terminology   *4*
References   *7*

1.   Identifying Families' Supports and Other Resources   9
LEE ANN JUNG

Why Does Ecology Matter?   *9*
Types of Family Supports, Resources, and Strengths   *10*
Conversations with Families about Supports   *12*
The Ecomap   *13*
Uses for the Ecomap   *19*
Conclusion   *22*
References   *22*
APPENDIX 1.1. Ecomap Checklist   25

2.   Assessing Families' Needs with the Routines-Based Interview   27
R. A. MCWILLIAM

The Need for a Functional Needs Assessment   *27*
Preparation for the RBI   *29*
Structure of the RBI   *30*
Documenting Results   *36*
Implementation Challenges and Solutions   *41*
Conclusion   *41*
References   *42*
APPENDIX 2.1. RBI Implementation Checklist   44
APPENDIX 2.2. RBI Report Form   48
APPENDIX 2.3. RBI–SAFER Combo   51

3. Community-Based Everyday Child Learning Opportunities   60

CARL J. DUNST, MELINDA RAAB, CAROL M. TRIVETTE, and JENNIFER SWANSON

Definition of Terms and Principles   62
Caregiver-Mediated Everyday Child Learning   63
Implementing and Practicing CMP   71
Conclusion   79
Acknowledgments   81
References   81
APPENDIX 3.1. Child Interests Checklist   88
APPENDIX 3.2. Everyday Community Learning Activity Checklist   89
APPENDIX 3.3. Increasing Everyday Child Learning Opportunities Checklist   90
APPENDIX 3.4. Caregiver Responsive Teaching Checklist   91
APPENDIX 3.5. Parent-Mediated Child Learning Evaluation Checklist   92

4. Coordinating Services with Families   93

MARY BETH BRUDER

The Research Foundation for Service Coordination   94
Coordinating the Performance of Evaluations and Assessments   96
Development, Review, and Evaluation of the IFSP   99
Assisting Families in Choosing Available Service Providers   103
Coordinating and Monitoring the Delivery of Available Services   106
Informing Families of the Availability of Advocacy Services   107
Coordinating with Medical and Health Providers   108
Facilitating the Development of a Transition Plan to Preschool Services   109
Using the Logic Model to Frame Evaluation   110
Conclusion   110
References   110
APPENDIX 4.1. Coordinating Evaluation and Assessments: First Contacts   112
APPENDIX 4.2. Coordinating and Implementing Evaluations and Assessments   114
APPENDIX 4.3. Facilitating and Participating in the Development, Review,
                         and Evaluation of the IFSP   116
APPENDIX 4.4. Assisting Families in Identifying Available Service Providers   118
APPENDIX 4.5. Coordinating and Monitoring the Delivery of Available Services   120
APPENDIX 4.6. Informing Families of the Availability of Advocacy Services   122
APPENDIX 4.7. Coordinating with Medical and Health Providers   123
APPENDIX 4.8. Facilitating the Development of a Transition Plan
                         to Preschool Services   125

5. Talking to Families   127

P. J. McWILLIAM

Create Opportunities for Informal Exchange   128
Acknowledge Child and Family Strengths   130
Solicit Parents' Opinions and Ideas   133
Seek Understanding   134
Demonstrate Caring for the Whole Family   137
Acknowledge and Respond to Feelings   140
Conclusion   142
References   143
APPENDIX 5.1. Talking to Families Checklist   144

6. **Working with Families from Diverse Backgrounds**   147
MARCI J. HANSON and ELEANOR W. LYNCH

What Is Diversity? 147
Developing and Enhancing Cross-Cultural Competence 154
Building Relationships with Families: Recognizing and Respecting Diversity 156
Partnering with Families to Develop and Address Goals 161
Achieving Responsive and Effective Services for Families from Diverse Backgrounds 168
Final Comments 170
References 170
APPENDIX 6.1. Checking the System for Cultural Competence 172
APPENDIX 6.2. Checking Program Implementation for Cultural Competence 173

7. **A Primary-Coach Approach to Teaming and Supporting Families**   175
in Early Childhood Intervention
M'LISA L. SHELDEN and DATHAN D. RUSH

Natural Learning Environment Practices 176
Coaching Families 177
Primary-Coach Approach to Teaming 181
Challenges to the Field 193
Conclusion 196
References 196
APPENDIX 7.1. Primary-Coach Approach to Teaming Checklist 201

8. **Support-Based Home Visiting**   203
R. A. MCWILLIAM

Home Visiting in Early Intervention 203
The Need for Guidelines for Home Visitors 207
A Framework for Home Visits 212
Functional Child Domains 218
Teaching Parents to Teach Their Children 219
Challenging Situations in Home Visiting 224
Conclusion 226
References 226
APPENDIX 8.1. Support-Based Home-Visiting Checklist 231
APPENDIX 8.2. Vanderbilt Home Visit Script 233

9. **Helping Families Address Challenging Behavior**   237
and Promote Social Development
LISE FOX

The Effect of Challenging Behavior on the Family 238
A Framework for Providing Support 239
Initiating the Conversation 240
Providing Information on Positive Parenting Techniques 244
Responding Effectively to Problem Behavior 247
Developing a Behavior Support Plan 249
Conclusion 253
References 254
APPENDIX 9.1. Home-Visiting Checklist: Addressing Challenging Behavior 257

Index   261

Introduction

R. A. MCWILLIAM

Working with Families of Young Children with Special Needs is designed for professionals in the trenches, local program administrators, and students. Readers who regularly work with, or soon will work with, families of children with disabilities from birth to 5 years of age will find practical information at a hitherto unprecedented level of detail. This book will be pertinent to professionals and students from a wide variety of disciplines, such as early childhood special educators, social workers, psychologists, occupational therapists, physical therapists, and speech–language pathologists.

PURPOSE OF THE BOOK

The purpose of this book is to present the most advanced thinking about appropriate methods of working with families of young children with disabilities. By "advanced thinking," I mean that the information is largely based on research or consistent with theory that has evolved over 35 years of intense growth in the field. Two of the most important theoretical and empirical bases for the practices are the *family-centered approach* and *social-support theory*. The former is rooted in family systems theory (Turnbull, Poston, Minnes, & Summers, 2007), ecobehavioral and developmental perspectives on how children learn (Greenwood, Carta, & Dawson, 2000; Vygotsky & Stone, 2005), and the consultative approach to how services work (McWilliam, 2003). The latter has implications for ways of serving families—in

1

a supportive manner (Turnbull et al., 2007)—as well as implications for making resources available to families (Dunst, Trivette, & Deal, 1994). By "appropriate methods," I mean the values and practices employed to carry out early intervention.

1. The first critical value is conducting interventions with children in the context of everyday routines rather than in sessions (Kashinath, Woods, & Goldstein, 2006).
2. The second value is working with families in a family-friendly manner rather than merely involving them in response to compliance requirements (Dunst, Trivette, & Hamby, 2007).
3. The third value is the concentration on family quality of life versus just on child competence (Lucyshyn et al., 2007).

Five practices are essential to my designation of appropriate methods: assessing informal and formal supports, assessing functional needs in everyday situations, coordinating services, using home visits to provide support, and consulting collaboratively with child care providers.

How Each Chapter Is Related to the Purpose

Each chapter is tied to the three values and five behaviors just described, which form the skeleton of the book around which the flesh and blood of actual strategies are formed.

In Chapter 1, Lee Ann Jung explains the use of ecomaps in assessing a family's ecology. A family's network of informal and formal supports is part of the family system. Examining the family's context is consistent with an ecobehavioral perspective as well as a social-support perspective. The ecomap is the specific practice for identifying resources available to the family.

In Chapter 2, I describe the Routines-Based Interview™, which assesses different family members' roles—a function consistent with family systems theory. The process is family friendly; explores resources available, especially informal ones; is obviously routines based; and includes a measure of family quality of life.

In Chapter 3, Carl Dunst, Melinda Raab, Carol Trivette, and Jennifer Swanson discuss serving families in the context of their communities. They define early intervention in part according to ecobehavioral and developmental principles about how children learn in routines. This chapter introduces the importance of "competency-enhancing outcomes that constitute measures of successful or effective early childhood intervention practices." The concept of caregiver-mediated everyday child learning that Dunst et al. discuss provides details on how children learn and how the implementation of caregiver-mediated practices is routines based.

In Chapter 4, Mary Beth Bruder reviews research showing that service coordination practices have been grouped in relational and participatory helpgiving, which is related to ways of serving families. The chapter discusses the use of an ecological framework for evaluating service coordination, consistent with the book's ecobehavioral perspective. Service coordination involves assisting families in choosing available service providers, which is connected to resources available to families.

In Chapter 5, P. J. McWilliam addresses professionals' interactional behaviors with families. She describes the importance of creating opportunities to have informal exchanges with families, typifying both the value of being family friendly and the principle of social support. Acknowledging child and family strengths recognizes the significance of the family's quality of life, and soliciting parents' opinions and seeking understanding are consistent with the consultative approach to families. Responding to feelings exemplifies both family friendliness and family quality of life.

Chapter 6 deals with diversity in early intervention, and Marci J. Hanson and Eleanor W. Lynch describe the importance of being family friendly with families from different cultures. Building relationships with families, recognizing and respecting diversity, is consistent with ways of serving families. Beliefs about family roles and views about children and childrearing are related to the consultative approach, and partnering with families to develop and address goals is related to social support. The authors describe special considerations in home-based services, which is discussed more fully in Chapter 8 on support-based home visits.

Teaming is discussed in Chapter 7, where M'Lisa L. Shelden and Dathan D. Rush define the primary-coach approach as one way to coordinate services. They describe natural learning environment practices, which illustrates one of the major points of this book—the distinction between routines and sessions. The parent-coaching section is related to support-based home visits, and the section on participation-based individualized family service plan (IFSP) outcomes is related both to assessing functional needs in everyday situations and the section on writing functional outcomes in Chapter 2.

In Chapter 8, I address quality home visits, describing the FACINATE model, which is connected to all the values and practices, but principally support-based home visits. The five key principles are consistent with all three values undergirding this book (already outlined), and the section on transdisciplinary service delivery is consistent with Chapter 7 in terms of practices involving the professional's role with the family (i.e., coach). The functional child domains featured in the chapter are related to the routines-based approach. Teaching parents to teach their children is consistent with how children learn.

Chapter 9 deals with challenging behaviors, and Lise Fox has described the effect of challenging behavior on the families in a way that is related to the concept of family quality of life. She has provided a framework for providing support, which is consistent with support-based home visits. Finally, providing information on positive parenting is related to how children learn.

BASIC THEMES

The three basic themes of the book are as follows:

1. How professionals should treat families (family friendliness).
2. What professionals should do with families (family centeredness).
3. Addressing family-level needs.

Although all chapters are consistent with the values and practices described earlier, they have some similarities and differences. Some chapters emphasize philosophical underpinnings (3, 4, 7, 9), whereas others emphasize procedures (1, 2, 5, 8). Some are closely related to planning (1, 2, 4), whereas others are closely related to intervention itself (3, 5, 6, 7, 8, 9).

VOICES IN THE CHAPTERS

Voices vary, and this variety has been preserved in part to provide diversity and in part to reflect the character of the different authors. These authors are luminaries in early intervention and early childhood special education and their individuality deserves to be maintained.

EARLY INTERVENTION/EARLY CHILDHOOD SPECIAL EDUCATION TERMINOLOGY

Rationale

Some terms are commonplace in early intervention/early childhood special education but not necessarily to the broader field of special education. The following brief glossary might help. Full descriptions of many of these terms are found within the book itself.

Brief Glossary

Collaborative consultation. This is a method of providing technical assistance in a manner involving *joint* decisions between the consultant and the consultee, such as between the therapist and the child care provider. It is applied most often in this book in the context of the provision of early childhood special education, occupational therapy, physical therapy, or speech–language to children in group care.

Consultative approach. This term describes early intervention aimed at the child's natural caregivers, such as parents and teachers, rather than directly at the child. It is used when the number of contact hours a professional has with the child is insufficient to make a difference in the child's learning or development, whereas the number of hours the caregivers have is sufficient to make a difference.

Contextually mediated practices. This term, coined by Carl Dunst et al. (see Chapter 3), is an intervention approach involving (1) the identification of children's interests and the everyday community and family activities that constitute the makeup of a child's life, (2) the selection of those activities that provide the best opportunities for interest-based learning, (3) an increase in child participation in interest-based, everyday learning opportunities, (4) the use of different interactional techniques for supporting and encouraging child competence, exploration, and mastery in the activities, and (5) an evaluation of the effectiveness of parent-mediated everyday child learning opportunities in terms of both child and parent benefits (Dunst, 2006; Dunst & Swanson, 2006).

Developmental perspectives. These perspectives refer to the practice of matching interactions, activities, and environments to the child's maturity or just above it, without establishing expectations more appropriate for older children. One characteristic of these perspectives can sometimes be a "constructivist" approach that deemphasizes direct instruction and emphasizes exploration and self-learning. This characteristic is generally repudiated by behaviorists.

Ecobehavioral perspectives. These perspectives refer to the practice of manipulating the interactions, activities, and environments to reinforce desired behavior and sometimes to withhold reinforcement for undesired behavior. One characteristic of these perspectives can sometimes be a structured approach that emphasizes the antecedents established by adults and deemphasizes independent initiations. This approach is generally repudiated by developmentalists.

Ecological framework. This framework stresses the impact of the social and sometimes the physical environment on children's learning. It can involve Bronfenbrenner's idea of systems moving outward from the child to include the family, the early intervention program, extended family, the neighborhood, and society. It can also refer to the behavioral idea that teaching young children involves manipulation of the environment.

Ecology. This word refers to the child's environment and does not have anything to do with being "green."

Ecomaps. These are pictures that professionals draw with families of families' informal, intermediate, and formal supports that show the strength of support each entity provides.

Family centeredness. This term refers to the way we treat families and what we attend to. The way we treat families consists of attitudes and behaviors such as positiveness, responsiveness, orientation to the whole family, friendliness, and sensitivity. What we attend to includes the needs of family members in addition to the child's, following the theory that what affects one family member has an impact on all other family members (i.e., family systems theory).

Family quality of life. This construct can involve a subjective appraisal by, in this case, the family. This would include families' satisfaction with their daily routines, for example. Another more objective dimension of family quality of life is access to essential resources, such as housing, food, a job, and medical care.

Family systems theory. As described above, this theory addresses the idea that a family is a dynamic system, whereby the behaviors and experiences of each family member affect the other members of the system.

Home visits. In this book, home visits are regular—usually weekly—visits by an early intervention professional to the family's home, to provide informational, emotional, and material support. A dated (although still prevalent) approach to home visits involved a professional "working" directly with the child in the home.

IFSP. The individualized family service plan (IFSP) is the central document around which early intervention for an individual family is built. It is the infant–toddler equivalent of the individualized education program (IEP).

Outcomes. In this book, this word generally refers to the goals established by the team, which includes families. It can also refer to overall or general results of early intervention, such as engagement, independence, and social relationships.

Primary-coach approach. "An established multidisciplinary team that meets regularly and selects one member as the primary coach who receives coaching from other team members, and uses coaching with parents and other care providers to support and strengthen their confidence and competence in promoting child learning and development and obtaining desired supports and resources in natural learning environments" (Shelden & Rush, 2007).

Routines. "Routines" is used here and in many early intervention contexts for frequently occurring times, events, and activities, such as waking up, meals, hanging out, bedtime at home, and circle, snack, centers, and outside play at child care or preschool.

Routines-Based Interview™. The Routines-Based Interview (RBI) is a specific procedure for conducting a semistructured clinical interview with families for the purposes of establishing a positive relationship, obtaining a rich and thick description of child and family functioning, and helping the family select a list of 6–10 functional outcomes.

Service coordination. Service coordination is mandated in the Individuals with Disabilities Education Improvement Act as a service that must be offered to families enrolling in Part C. It is designed to ensure that families have access to resources, including services; this means the service coordinator is responsible for the development of the IFSP. Service coordinators also ensure that family-level needs not addressed by other providers are met and ensure that the various services are coordinated.

Service providers. "Service providers" refers to professionals working with children and families. In situations where service coordinators only do service coordination, "service provider" refers to interventionists.

Social support. Social support is the provision of emotional encouragement or material help by other people or agencies, such as formal supports (professionals, agencies), informal supports (kith and kin), or intermediate supports (recreational activities, work, religious affiliations).

Supports. "Supports" is used as a generic term to include those activities, interventions, or programs that might be offered to families in early intervention. Often, it is used instead of "services," to make the point that resources beyond formal services are appropriate.

Transdisciplinary service delivery. This model of service delivery involves the use of one person who addresses areas traditionally covered by his or her own discipline as well as areas traditionally covered by people from other disciplines. It therefore involves "role release" by people from other disciplines and "role acceptance" by the transdisciplinary service provider. It differs from multidisciplinary service delivery, which involves multiple professionals each independently addressing only his or her area of expertise, and interdisciplinary service delivery, which involves multiple professionals addressing their own areas of expertise but communicating with each other.

REFERENCES

Dunst, C. J. (2006). Parent-mediated everyday child learning opportunities: I. Foundations and operationalization. *CASEinPoint, 2*(2), 1–10.

Dunst, C. J., & Swanson, J. (2006). Parent-mediated everyday child learning opportunities: II. Methods and procedures. *CASEinPoint, 2*(11), 1–19.

Dunst, C. J., Trivette, C. M., & Deal, A. G. (1994). Resource-based family-centered intervention practices. In C. J. Dunst, C. M. Trivette, & A. G. Deal (Eds.), *Supporting and strengthening families: Methods, strategies and practices* (pp. 140–151). Cambridge, MA: Brookline Books.

Dunst, C. J., Trivette, C. M., & Hamby, D. W. (2007). Meta-analysis of family-centered helpgiving practices research. *Mental Retardation and Developmental Disabilities Research Reviews, 13*(4), 370–378.

Greenwood, C. R., Carta, J. J., & Dawson, H. (2000). Ecobehavioral Assessment Systems Software (EBASS): A system for observation in education settings. In T. Thompson, D. Felce, & F. Symons (Eds.), *Behavioral observation: Technology and applications in developmental disabilities* (pp. 229–251). Baltimore: Brookes.

Kashinath, S., Woods, J., & Goldstein, H. (2006). Enhancing generalized teaching strategy use in daily routines by parents of children with autism. *Journal of Speech, Language, and Hearing Research, 49*, 466–485.

Lucyshyn, J. M., Albin, R. W., Horner, R. H., Mann, J. C., Mann, J. A., & Wadsworth, G. (2007). Family implementation of positive behavior support for a child with autism: Longitudinal, single-case, experimental, and descriptive replication and extension. *Journal of Positive Behavior Interventions, 9*(3), 131–150.

McWilliam, R. A. (2003). The primary-service-provider model for home- and community-based services. *Psicologia: Revista da Associacao Portuguesa Psicologia, 17*(1), 115–135.

Turnbull, A. P., Poston, D. J., Minnes, P., & Summers, J. A. (2007). Providing supports and services that enhance a family's quality of life. In I. Brown & M. Percy (Eds.), *A comprehensive guide to intellectual and developmental disabilities* (pp. 561–571). Baltimore: Brookes.

Vygotsky, L. S., & Stone, L. R. (2005). Appendix. *Journal of Russian and East European Psychology, 43*(2), 90–97.

CHAPTER 1

Identifying Families' Supports and Other Resources

LEE ANN JUNG

Understanding a family's ecology (e.g., who makes up the family, what supports and resources they have, what they do, what they enjoy) is a critical piece to designing intervention that is *meaningful* and *relevant*. As early intervention professionals plan the intervention for a child with special needs, they have a wealth of developmental strategies available—strategies that promote child competence. But choosing the direction and methods for intervention is much more complex than matching an intervention to a need for a skill. Because children each have unique experiences made up of their daily routines and family context, intervention must not only match a need for a skill, but also fit well within the child's unique family situation. Furthermore, many of the interventions and supports early intervention professionals provide are not even related to developmental skills. Supports are often designed instead to meet family-level priorities. The purpose of this chapter is to describe procedures for creating a picture of a family's supports, called an ecomap, as a means for talking about and building upon a family's ecology as a foundation for early intervention supports.

WHY DOES ECOLOGY MATTER?

For children with disabilities, we know that in order to design intervention that is effective, we must have a clear grasp of the child's current developmental skills. At first glance, understanding a family's ecology may seem much less important than understanding the child's present level of development. After all, if we understand where a child is developmentally, and we understand what specific interventions correspond with the different areas of development, we should be able to design effective intervention programs. Right? Well, that's part of the story. Ecological systems theory (Bronfenbrenner, 1979) reminds us, though, that children develop within a *context* of environmental influences that have direct and indirect effects on them. Every child's experience is different, and there are numerous different collections of experiences that can effectively promote development (Dunst, 2007). To truly understand the course of children's development, and create a plan to promote their development, we have to understand the perceptions, values, beliefs, supports, resources, and daily lives that make up the context of their development (Bernheimer & Keogh, 1995).

Ecological systems theory also contends that there are certain environmental influences that have the potential for greater *direct* effect than others. Clearly, the natural caregivers who spend more time with a child have the greatest opportunity for direct effect on the child's development. By contrast, those who spend relatively small portions of time with the child (such as early intervention professionals) have ample opportunity for *indirect effect* but fewer opportunities for direct influence than do the caregivers. In part because of this difference in opportunities for direct influence on development, the field of early intervention has grown in the past decade to involve much more than providing developmental services to children. In fact, the focus in many ways has shifted away from providing developmental services to children toward providing and coordinating supports to the people in the child's life (Turnbull, Blue-Banning, Turbiville, & Park, 1999). In this way, those who have the greatest opportunity to make a direct impact are given the information and supports they need to be able to do so. And those who have few opportunities to have direct influence instead concentrate their efforts on supporting those who do.

Because the focus has moved from supporting the child to supporting the family, *how* supports are provided is just as important as *what* supports are provided. In order to carefully design intervention that fits families' lives, early intervention professionals need an understanding of the family, its informal and formal resources, and its interacting social networks. To this end, understanding the family's ecology is as important to designing intervention as understanding the child's development.

TYPES OF FAMILY SUPPORTS, RESOURCES, AND STRENGTHS

When discussing supports and resources with families, considering the *categories* of support that are available can help early intervention professionals and families easily see which areas are relative strengths and in which categories additional resources may be needed. For example, a family may have an extensive network of families and friends who are helpful with child care and provide a social support. But the family may have relatively few financial resources. Having this understanding can guide the early intervention professionals to concentrate on linking the family to financial supports they may not have accessed. Supports can be divided into three categories: *emotional, material,* or *informational* (McWilliam & Scott, 2001).

Emotional Support

Emotional support is important for all families, but especially so for families experiencing any kind of psychological distress (Baider, Ever-Hadani, Goldzweig, Wygoda, & Peretz, 2003), such as many families who have a child with disabilities do. Families usually receive much of their needed emotional support through their informal social networks—their family and friends (Waltrowicz, Ames, McKenzie, & Flicker, 1996). Families who are lacking a sense of emotional support can feel isolated (Aoun, 2004; van Teijlingen, Friend, & Kamal, 2001), hopeless (Cattell, 2001), or depressed (Soothill et al., 2001; van Teijlingen et al., 2001; Ray & Street, 2005). An important part of emotional support for some families is parent-to-parent support. The early intervention professional may give the family information on a support group or the contact information for another parent who lives nearby. Being able to identify and use sources of emotional support is fundamental to a family's feeling of confidence, sense of control, and self-worth (Cattell, 2001; Ray & Street, 2005). Early intervention professionals and others in the family's formal support systems also provide direct emotional support through listening and responding to the family, being positive and strengths oriented, and through general warmth and friendliness.

Material Support

Material support includes access to financial and physical resources families need for functioning and progress toward their goals. Examples of material support include food, shelter, clothing, diapers, medical equipment, child care, toys, and so forth. If a family's most basic needs such as housing and food are not met, the family is less able to focus on higher-level needs (Maslow, 1954), such as their child's development and intervention. Examples of ways early intervention professionals can provide material support include linking a family to a community resource, such as a food or diaper bank, providing assistive technology, or helping a family to access medical benefits.

Informational Support

Informational support includes resources to meet a family's need to know and understand. Most commonly, family members want information in four areas: (1) their child's disability, (2) services that are available, (3) general child development, and 4) strategies to use with their child (McWilliam & Scott, 2001). Some families may have little information on these topics and prefer to receive much of this information from early intervention professionals. Other families may instead seek out information first from friends, family, or other resources, such as the Internet, and prefer that early intervention professionals instead serve to clarify or provide guidance on the information they find. Examples of other kinds of information practitioners might provide are ideas for recreation opportunities, types of equipment or toys that might be useful, or options for child care in the community.

Formal or Informal Support

Within the above three categories of support, each can also be characterized as *formal* or *informal*. Formal supports are made up of people and groups of people or agencies that are formally organized for the purpose of responding to particular family needs (Dunst, Trivette, & Deal, 1988). Examples of formal supports include health care providers, medical specialists, therapists, hospitals, and early intervention programs. Informal supports are those people and groups that became a part of families' lives for reasons other than their child's disability. Examples of informal support include extended family, neighbors, friends, churches, and recreational clubs (Dunst et al., 1988). Identifying what informal supports a family has is an important consideration in deciding what additional formal supports might be needed. Evidence shows that families find support most helpful when it is a part of the informal social support network (Dunst, 2000; National Center for Family Support, n.d.). The people and places where families turn in the most difficult times are often this network of informal supports (McDonald, Kysela, Drummand, Alexander, Enns, & Chambers, 1999). These informal and natural supports should be the primary means for strengthening and supporting families. (Dunst, 2000; Hobbs et al., 1984). By determining which supports are a natural part of a family's informal support network, early intervention professionals can choose formal supports only when necessary and in a way that complements rather than supplant existing informal supports and community resources.

CONVERSATIONS WITH FAMILIES ABOUT SUPPORTS

Because information on natural family resources, strengths, and other supports is important to the entire individualized education program (IEP) and individualized family service plan (IFSP) planning process, identifying this information in the earliest meetings with a family is important. During the first conversations with early intervention professionals, families gain ideas about what they can expect from early intervention and how early intervention supports will look. They may be asking, "Will the supports focus on my child? Or do they involve my entire family? Will this be a formal, ultraprofessional relationship with an expert and me? Or will it be casual and include relaxed, comfortable conversation? Does the team seem confident in my abilities and contributions as a parent? Or do they seem to think I have a lot to learn in order to support my child?" Without ever directly addressing the topic, early intervention professionals can give families a sense of how they fit into the team. Clearly, we want families to know that early intervention supports are aimed at the entire family and build upon the strengths, resources, and supports already available to the family.

Although early intervention professionals are likely to see the value in gaining quality information on natural family resources and supports during beginning meetings, they are often challenged with timeline and paperwork pressures. Many agencies and schools require a great deal of paperwork to be completed with families initially to meet timelines for IFSPs or IEPs that are required for children who qualify for early intervention or special education services, respectively. These paperwork requirements can quickly shift any early intervention professional's attention away from the family-centered *process* to the *products* that must be completed. This pressure can lead teams to choose traditional checklists or questionnaires without an accompanying interview to acquire the required information on family resources and supports. Or teams may wait to ask about resources and supports until the day of the IFSP or IEP meeting, when decisions about intervention are to be made. Unfortunately, when these more rushed methods are used, the supports teams' lists can begin to look the same (e.g., "good housing," "good transportation," "adequate medical care," "good child care" [Jung & Baird, 2003]. Such lists of supports do not provide meaningful information for developing intervention that is relevant to families.

So how, given pressure of IFSP and IEP timelines, can early intervention professionals facilitate meaningful conversations about resources, strengths, and supports? Professionals need a simple, time-efficient method for identifying family resources and supports. Rather than depending solely on checklists or rushing through discussion the day of the formal IFSP or IEP meeting, early intervention professionals and families need to be able to have a high-quality discussion on resources and supports that will be useful. These conversations should contribute to planning systematically the best way to use formal early intervention supports. Developing ecomaps is one such method that gives professionals the opportunity to transform the often sterile feeling of traditional questionnaire-style intake paperwork into a natural-feeling, more casual conversation. Yet the structure of the ecomap facilitates a time-efficient process that can be completed in 20–30 minutes.

THE ECOMAP

An *ecomap* is a diagram of an individual family's connections, resources, and supports, and the relative strength of each one (Hartman, 1978; Olsen, Dudley-Brown,

& McMullen, 2004). The ecomap was developed by Ann Hartman in 1975 as part of her practice in social work at the University of Michigan (Hartman, 1995). Hartman, drawing on the theory of human ecology, developed the ecomap as a tool to represent the social relationships and social systems that people have created. Originally, the ecomap was a tool to guide social workers' reflections on a family's relationships without the family present. Its value as an interview tool, though, was quickly recognized (Hartman, 1995), and its utility, it has been used in many fields, including social work (e.g., Hartman, 1995; Early et al., 2000), nursing, (e.g., MacDonald & Callery, 2008; Ray & Street, 2005; Rempel, Neufeld, & Kushner, 2007), and psychology (e.g., Christiansen, Wittenborn, Kavakurt, Abdullah, & Zhang, 2007). Across disciplines and purposes, the visual impact of the ecomap is its clearest utility (Hartman, 1995).

Ecomaps also provide a springboard to further conversation about how various relationships came about or how the nature of relationships has changed over time. Because the process involves conversation and reflection, it is much more likely to foster rapport than are traditional surveys and scales. Hartman (1995) found that through the use of the ecomap, unlike a traditional interview, families did not feel threatened by the feeling of being judged during assessment of family supports. Instead, families saw the professionals as wanting to gain an idea of what it was like to walk in their shoes.

Because the process results in a picture, the people in and connections of a family are literally visible, allowing them to see their family in a new way. The ecomap can be a comfort to some families. They commonly make reflective comments, such as, "Wow! I didn't realize I had that much!" or, "Gee, I never saw myself like that before!" (Hartman, 1995, p. 117). Still others might find the map validating and might remark, "Now I see why I'm so stressed. Almost everything flows *away* from me." Most families enjoy the process of creating their family ecomap and like to have a copy (Hartman, 1995). An example of an ecomap for the family of a 3-year-old who receives preschool special education and related services is presented in Figure 1.1.

There are three ways described in the literature to facilitate an ecomap: (1) the practitioner can construct the ecomap from his or her perspective without family involvement; (2) the family can construct the ecomap with assistance from the practitioner; or (3) it can be a collaborative process between the practitioner and the family (Hartman, 1995). For early intervention, the collaborative option has distinct advantages for identifying family resources and supports. Because IFSPs, in particular, are built upon family strengths, resources, and priorities, the perspective of the family is the only one that matters. The practitioner's view of the family resources and relationships are irrelevant. Although the family's taking the lead would have the advantage of being completely family driven, because the ecomap should be used in the initial contacts with families, the family might not be comfortable taking on such a role. For these reasons, I describe a collaborative process for creating the ecomap.

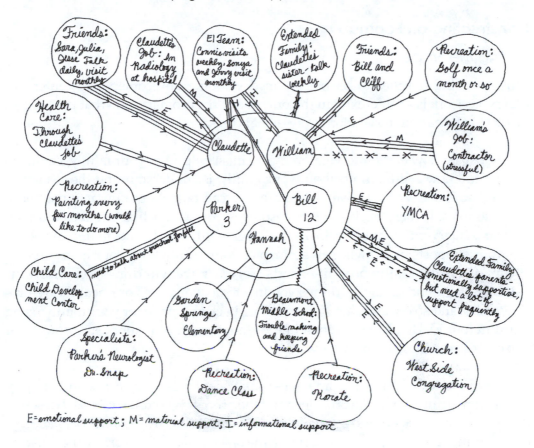

FIGURE 1.1. Example of an ecomap.

Getting Ready to Develop an Ecomap

The ecomap is a simple tool to create and, thus, requires little practice and preparation. One of the best ways to prepare the development of an ecomap with a family is to map your own family first (Hartman, 1995). After doing this and then practicing with friends or colleagues, early intervention professionals usually feel confident in trying it with a family for whom they are providing services (Hartman, 1995). Choosing a family with whom you already have an established relationship might be a good way to begin using it with the families you serve. To prepare, you will need a large piece of blank paper with no lines. Many people find that larger than 8.5″ × 11″ is preferable. Some prefer the 11″ × 17″ size because it is large enough to provide plenty of room for drawing, yet can be folded in half and stored in a standard file or record folder. Some people like to use a photocopied blank ecomap with circles and categories already in place to save time (Hartman, 1995). If a blank map is used, it is a good idea to leave some circles with no category to allow for individual family variation. I prefer to draw the circles of the ecomap during the process so that it is completely unique to the individual family.

Constructing an Ecomap

Setting the Stage

When inviting families to participate in developing an ecomap, early intervention professionals should explain the purpose of the ecomap and what the process involves. The early intervention professional can say:

> "To decide how early intervention can be most helpful to your family, I'd like to get to know a little more about your family. By understanding the resources and supports you all have as a family, we can talk about how you use those resources, if there are any other resources you would like to have, and how early intervention might help. If it's all right with you, I'd like to find out about your supports by drawing an ecomap of your family with your help. An ecomap is like a family portrait of sorts. Together, we will draw circles for your friends, extended family, things you like to do, your job, your health care providers, and so on, and then connect those back to a circle for your family using different kinds of lines, depending on how much of a support, resource, or even stress these each are."

Next, ask if the family has any questions and whether they are willing to participate, ensuring that families understand the process is voluntary. Next, I describe the three major tasks of the ecomap process: identifying *people and social networks*, determining *relationships*, and describing the *type and flow of support*. A checklist for creating the ecomap is presented in Appendix 1.1.

People and Social Networks

The interview begins with asking about the people living in the household. Each person should have his or her own circle. Inside each person's circle, it can be helpful to write the person's age (Hartman, 1995). I often write the ages of only the children in the household. In the ecomap example in Figure 1.1, Claudette is the mother, William the father, and Parker, Hannah, and Bill, their three children. Once each member of the household has a circle, draw a circle around the family unit.

Next, surround the family circle with other circles that represent the people and systems in their social network. A list of the common support categories available to families is found in Table 1.1. The table is sequenced from informal, closest supports at the top to most formal and distant supports at the bottom. Because of the importance of informal, natural supports, ask about these first. Once the closest support networks are discussed (e.g., family and friends), the interviewer can then move to those supports that are next closest (e.g., recreational activities, work), doing so until all supports are discussed. Organizing the space by support type makes the relative number of each type of support more clear. For example, you might place all of the informal support circles across the top, all of the formal support circles across the bottom, and those that are in between along the sides.

TABLE 1.1. Sources of Family Support

Category of support	Examples
Nuclear family	Spouse or partner, children, others in the household
Kinship	Aunts, uncles, cousins, grandparents
Informal network	Friends, neighbors, friends from church and work
Social organizations and activities	Church, social clubs, recreational activities
Generic professionals	Primary health care provider, child care, school
Specialists	Early intervention professionals, therapists, medical specialists
Policymakers	Agency directors, legislators, school boards

Note. Adapted from Dunst, Trivette, and Deal (1988). Copyright 1988 by Brookline Book. Adapted by permission.

Throughout the interview the early intervention professional can give examples of systems such as friends, family, recreation, church, work, school, child care, and health care to prompt the family to think about common systems. For example, to facilitate discussion on friends, the professional might say, "Many people list their friends on the ecomap. We can list both friends of the whole family as well as friends specific to one person in your family. Do you have friends that we can list?" In addition to the example categories found in Table 1.1, families might think of other categories that are unique to them. For each category, draw a circle, and in the circle write the category name (e.g., friends, extended family, work friends) and/or any other details such as names or descriptive phrases that can clarify the nature of the relationship or support. You can have multiple circles of the same category. For example, if each parent attends a different church, you would have two "church" circles, each with a different name.

Determining Relationships

Once social networks are identified, the early intervention professional guides conversation on the *relationships* that connect the family or family members to each network. The American Heritage Dictionary (2000) refers to the word *relationship* as "a particular type of connection existing between people related to or having dealings with each other." On the ecomap, lines are drawn to represent the relationship between the family and each of the people or social networks that have been included on the map. Lines can connect a system to the family as a unit or can connect to an individual in the family, indicating whether there is a relationship to the entire family or to an individual. For example, Bill and Cliff, in the example ecomap, are William's friends and are connected directly to his circle. Church, on the other hand, is a resource and support for the whole family and is therefore connected to the circle for the family unit. To indicate the nature or strength of relationships between the family and the people and systems in their environment, several types of lines described by Hartman (1995) are used. *Solid lines* represent positive or significant relationships or support, *dotted or dashed lines* indicate a weak, fragile, or questionable connection, and a *jagged or hashed line* is used to indicate relationships characterized by stress or conflict.

Although these three types of lines were found sufficient for analytic purposes in the field of social work, when used as a means to facilitate interviews, families and social workers viewed this as constraining (Hartman, 1995). I also found this constraining and needed a way to vary the solid lines to indicate *how* positive or strong the relationship was. Like Hodge (2005), I think it useful to vary the number of solid lines indicating degree of strength, with more lines indicating stronger relationships or support. Some people describe varying the thickness of line (Wright & Leahey, 2000) with strength, but I found that varying the number of lines both (1) provides clearer information on a family's comparison of strength of support in their lives, and (2) is easier and quicker. Although Ray and Street (2005) limited the range of lines used on the ecomap to one to three, I have found that leaving this open allows the family to distinguish level of support to whatever extent they like.

Once the line is drawn from a system to the family or family member, details can be added along the line (Hartman, 1995) that describe the type of support for each relationship. Because early intervention should be about mobilizing, coordinating, and providing material, emotional, and informational support (McWilliam & Scott, 2001), I like to indicate the type or types of support directly on lines. I use abbreviations: "M" for material, "E" for emotional, and "I" for informational. In this way, the family and I get a visual of how much of each type of support is available.

In the example ecomap in Figure 1.1, Claudette listed Sarah, Julia, and Jesse as her closest friends. She drew five lines to them. On the line we wrote "E" because they provide one another with the emotional support of close friendship. Also, by using only an abbreviation, there is additional room for comments on the line if needed. Claudette and William were very pleased with Parker's child care center but knew that the preschool classroom at Garden Springs Elementary was an option for fall. Even though their daughter, Hannah, goes to Garden Springs, they didn't know much about the preschool classroom and weren't sure they wanted to transition there. On the line between child care and Parker, the interviewer noted that they needed to talk about the option of transitioning to the preschool classroom in the fall.

Flow of Support

For each relationship line (or set of lines), arrows can be drawn to indicate the direction of resources, energy, or interest. Arrows can be pointed in both directions for one relationship, indicating flow in and flow out. Different types of lines can even be used for a single relationship to distinguish the strength and type of resources flowing in from strength and type of resources flowing out. For example, there might be a solid line with arrows away from the family and a dashed line with arrows toward the family. This would mean, as Claudette's parents on the example ecomap in Figure 1.1, that the family is providing a lot of support or energy, but the support coming to the family is weak or questionable.

USES FOR THE ECOMAP

Intervention Planning

The information generated from developing an ecomap is an important foundation to intervention planning for a child with disabilities. Any intervention that is designed must work well not only for the child, but also for the family. Take, for example, the skill of walking over uneven surfaces. There are many ways to intervene to support the development of this skill. I imagine that right now you can think of 10 activities that would promote a child's ability to walk across uneven surfaces. But not every way we can imagine would work equally well for every family. Instead, we would need to consider the uneven surfaces that are a part of that family's life. Where in that family's life does the child need that skill? And what resources are available in his or her home and places he or she frequent to promote that skill? By answering questions like these, in part through the ecomap process, teams can choose methods that are relevant for families. The team can design intervention that the family is comfortable implementing, makes use of the resources families have, and fits well within what great things the family already does or wants to do.

Determining the Need for Additional Supports

Although the primary focus of the ecomap is identifying supports and resources, gaps in these might also become evident. Coordinating, mobilizing, and providing supports is an important part of families' ability to care for their children in ways that enhance child development and family outcomes (Dunst, Trivette, & Deal, 1994). We can look back to the work by Maslow (1954) to know that for early intervention professionals, the first priorities are addressing the more basic needs of a family. Because of the relative effects of informal versus formal supports (Dunst et al., 1988) we also know that early intervention professionals can be most supportive by seeking to meet needs first with informal, rather than formal supports. Figure 1.2 is a model practitioners can use to guide them through assessing the most basic needs first, and matching needs to informal supports second.

For example, if a family's food, shelter, safety, and health needs are met, the next most basic need might be a mother's desire to talk to someone about her child and family. She might be in an isolated area without accessible transportation. Thus,

Family Needs		Sources of Support		
		Informal ————————————————————————→ Formal		
Basic	Food	Spouse/partner, friends, family, neighbors; friends from church and work	Recreational and social clubs; church or other religious organizations; service clubs; child care; school	Early intervention program; therapists; health care providers; medical specialists; hospital
	Shelter			
	Safety			
	Health			
	Belongingness			
	Communication/ mobility			
	Education			
	Spirituality			
	Autonomy			
Higher level	Generativity			

FIGURE 1.2. Matching family needs to supports available.

her opportunities for friendship and social interaction might be limited. Although the formal supports of early intervention will in fact provide some of the emotional support she would like to have, a better match would be to research the available natural supports that might help meet this need. This could include access to transportation and social groups in the community, or possibly linking her with other mothers to begin a relationship that might be maintained through frequent phone contact and occasional evening social opportunities. Table 1.2 includes questions Hartman and Laird (1983) have suggested that may be used as they discuss the need for support.

Determining Goals for the Future

As a variation of the ecomap, professionals can, in addition to the original map of current support, create with families future ecomaps that show how the family would like for its ecology to change. Early intervention professionals can consider a number of questions when beginning conversations about how and if the family would like to see their ecomap change. A quicker version of a future ecomap, space permitting, is to use a different color ink or a pencil to include the desired changes and additions on the original ecomap. Or the family can simply discuss changes they would like to see while the interviewer takes notes. The needs for support the

TABLE 1.2. Questions to Consider When Reviewing an Ecomap to Begin Intervention Planning

1. Does the family have sufficient income for basic needs?
2. Is there adequate food and shelter?
3. Does the family feel safe in the neighborhood?
4. Can the family gain access to preventative health care and medical resources?
5. Does the family have needed communication and transportation resources to gain access to other needed resources and supports?
6. Does the family have positive relationships with family, friends, or community organizations?
7. Are family members a part of any group activities?
8. Is the family able to share cultural and other types of values with those around them?
9. Is the family satisfied with the educational opportunities for the children and adults?
10. Do the family members work? Are they satisfied with their work?
11. Are family members able to master new experiences or contribute to something in ways that make them proud or fulfilled?

Note. Adapted from Hartman and Laird (1983, p. 166). Copyright 1983 by the authors. Adapted by permission.

family identifies or areas on the map they would like to strengthen can be used in the development of goals for IEPs and IFSPs.

Evaluating Outcomes and Measuring Change

An ecomap can be saved and then revisited at a later date, such as when reviewing an IFSP or IEP, to look for changes in relationships and supports. Hartman (1995) found that when people reviewed their ecomaps from an earlier interview, they were interested in the changes. Some wanted to add people and other supports they had forgotten, and others modified the lines to indicate changes in relationships and types of support. Hartman described several instances in which a family member *initiated* this review and change of the actual map. They wanted to see on the map how an important relationship in their life had changed. By modifying the ecomap or constructing a new one, changes in the family's overall supports can be seen immediately. Families might be more likely to demonstrate this level of interest in their review of resources and supports with an ecomap than if a review of supports is conducted through more traditional surveys or scales.

Clarifying the Nature of Early Intervention

Reviewing an ecomap also affords an opportunity to discuss the nature of early intervention supports that can be expected. In the example, Parker's mother drew three lines from the early intervention team. Notice that the lines connect to the caregivers and the oldest sibling, not to Parker. By discussing who is really being supported as shown by the visual information in the ecomap, we decided that the lines didn't make sense drawn to Parker. This can be a powerful visual to again reinforce team understanding of early intervention as a family-centered support and not services model. Also, by asking parents and caregivers about their families, friends, and community supports, providers clearly demonstrate that early intervention supports the whole family, not just the child.

CONCLUSION

The ecomap is an effective and efficient method that early intervention professionals can use to assess the ecology with a family and incorporate this important information into a comprehensive plan for intervention and support. Although having information about the current development of a child with disabilities is certainly a necessary part of planning intervention, understanding the ecology of the child's family is equally important. This ecology is a key piece of the puzzle that is necessary to designing intervention and coordinating supports that are meaningful and relevant to the family. With this information, early intervention professionals can go beyond matching intervention strategies to skills identified on a traditional developmental assessment. Instead, information on family connections, resources, and supports provide them with much of what they need to be able to design with families an intervention that responds to their entire family's needs and makes use of the best resources and supports available. Further, having a clear understanding of the family's resources, supports, and strengths, early intervention professionals can design more comprehensive intervention that meets the developmental needs not only of the child but also of the entire family.

REFERENCES

The American Heritage Dictionary of the English Language (4th ed.). (2000). Boston: Houghton Mifflin.

Aoun, S. (2004, May). *The hardest thing we have ever done: The social impact of caring for terminally ill people in Australia: Full report of the National Inquiry into the Social Impact of Caring for Terminally Ill People.* Canberra, Australia: Palliative Care Australia.

Baider, L. Ever-Hadani, P., Goldzweig, G., Wygoda, M., & Peretz, T. (2003). Is perceived family support a relevant variable in psychological distress: A sample of prostate and breast cancer couples. *Journal of Psychosomatic Research, 55,* 1–8.

Bernheimer, L. P., & Keogh, B. K. (1995). Weaving interventions into the fabric of everyday life: An approach to family assessment. *Topics in Early Childhood Special Education, 15,* 415–433.

Bronfenbrenner, U. (1979). *The ecology of human development.* Cambridge, MA: Harvard University Press.

Cattell, V. (2001). Poor people, poor places, and poor health: The mediating role of social networks and social capital. *Social Science and Medicine, 52,* 1501–1516.

Christiansen, A., Wittenborn, A., Karakurt, G., Abdullah, S., & Zhang, C. (2007). Exploring relationships: An eco-map activity for adult survivors of incest. In L. L. Hecker & C. F. Sori (Eds.), *The therapist's notebook: Vol. 2. More homework, handouts, and activities for use in psychotherapy* (pp. 159–168). New York: Haworth Press.

Dunst, C. J. (2000). Revisiting "rethinking early intervention." *Topics in Early Childhood Special Education, 20,* 95–104.

Dunst, C. J. (2007). Early intervention for infants and toddlers with developmental disabilities. In S. L. Odom, R. H. Horner, M. E. Snell, & J. Blacher (Eds.), *Handbook of developmental disabilities* (pp. 531–551). New York: Guilford Press.

Dunst, C. J., Trivette, C. M., & Deal, A. (1988). *Enabling and empowering families: Principles and guidelines for practice.* Cambridge, MA: Brookline Books.

Dunst, C. J., Trivette, C. M., & Deal, A. G. (1994). Resource-based family-centered intervention practices. In C. J. Dunst, C. M. Trivette, & A. G. Deal (Eds.), *Supporting and strengthening families: Methods, strategies and practices* (pp. 140–151). Cambridge, MA: Brookline Books.

Early, B. P., Smith, E. D., Todd, L., & Beem, T. (2000). The needs and supportive networks of the dying: An assessment instrument and mapping procedure for hospice patients. *American Journal of Hospice and Palliative Care, 17,* 87–96.

Hartman, A. (1978) Diagrammatic assessment of family relationships. *Social Casework, 59,* 465–476.

Hartman, A. (1995). Diagrammatic assessment in family relationships. *Families in Society, 76,* 111–122.

Hartman, A., & Laird, J. (1983). *Family-centered social work practice.* New York: Free Press.

Hodge, D. R. (2005). Developing a spiritual assessment toolbox: A discussion of the strengths and limitations of five different assessment methods. *Health and Social Work, 30*(4), 314–323.

Jung, L. A., & Baird, S. M. (2003). Effects of service coordinator variables on individualized family service plans. *Journal of Early Intervention, 25,* 206–218.

MacDonald, H., & Callery, P. (2008, March). Parenting children requiring complex care: A journey through time. *Child: Care, Health, and Development, 34,* 207–213.

Maslow, A. H. (1954). *Motivation and personality.* New York: Harper & Row.

McDonald, L., Kysela, G. M., Drummond, L., Alexander, J., Enns, R., & Chambers, J. (1999). Individual family planning using the family adaptation model. *Developmental Disabilities Bulletin, 27*(1), 16–29.

McWilliam, R. A., & Scott, S. (2001). A support approach to early intervention: A three-part framework. *Infants and Young Children, 13*(4), 55–66.

National Center for Family Support. (n.d.) *Essential features of family support programs.* Retrieved January 11, 2006, from *www.familysupport-hsri.org/resources/r_essentials-2.html.*

Olsen, S. J., Dudley-Brown, S., & McMullen, P. (2004). The case for blending pedigrees, genograms, and ecomaps. Nursing's contribution to the "big picture." *Nursing and Health Sciences, 6*(4), 295–308.

Ray, R. A., & Street, A. F. (2005). Ecomapping: An innovative research tool for nurses. *Journal of Advanced Nursing, 50,* 545–552.

Rempel, G., Neufeld, A., & Kushner, K. (2007, November). Interactive use of genomes and ecomaps in family caregiving research. *Journal of Family Nursing, 13,* 403–419.

Soothill, K., Morris, S. M., Harman, J. C., Francis, B., Thomas, C., & McIllmurray, M. B. (2001). Informal carers of cancer patients: What are their unmet social needs? *MB Health and Social Care in the Community, 9,* 464–475.

Turnbull, A. P., Blue-Banning, M., Turbiville, V., & Park, J. (1999). From parent education to partnership education: A call for transformed focus. *Topics in Early Childhood Special Education, 19,* 164–172.

van Teijlingen, E. R., Friend, E., & Kamal, A. D. (2001). Service use and needs of people with motor neurone disease and their carers in Scotland. *Health and Social Care in the Community, 9,* 397–403.

Waltrowicz, W., Ames, D., McKenzie, S., & Flicker, L. (1996). Burden and stress on relatives (informal carers) of dementia suffers in psychogeriatric nursing homes. *Australian Journal on Ageing, 15,* 115–118.

Wright, L. M. & Leahey, M. (2000). *Nurses and families: A guide to family assessment and intervention* (3rd ed.). Philadelphia: Davis.

Ecomap Checklist

Interviewer: _____ Date: _____

Observer: _____

Did the interviewer . . .	✓ ✗ ? NA	Notes
Getting started		
1. Explain the purpose of the ecomap to the family member?		
2. Explain to the family that their participation is voluntary?		
3. Begin with the people living in the house?		
4. Include ages of each child?		
5. Draw a circle around the whole family?		
Identifying social networks		
6. Prompt the family to think about common social systems from those closest to those farthest away?		
a. Kinship (blood and marriage relatives)		
b. Informal network (friends, neighbors, church friends, work friends)		
c. Social organizations (church, social clubs, recreational activities/organizations, service organizations)		
d. Generic professionals (primary health care provider, hospital, child care provider, school)		
e. Specialists (special instructor/educator, therapists, medical specialists)		

(cont.)

✓ = done at a satisfactory level; ✗ = not done; ? = perhaps done or done but perhaps not at a satisfactory level; NA = not appropriate (e.g., ran out of time).

Did the interviewer . . .	✓ ✗ ? NA	Notes
7. For each circle, write the category or other details as appropriate?		
Determining relationships		
8. Explain to family the line types and how they are used (optional)?		
9. Begin with closest support source and for each prompt discussion on the nature of support, draw appropriate line (solid, dashed, jagged)?		
10. For relationships described as positive, discuss the strength of relationship and indicates so by varying the number or thickness of lines?		
11. For each relationship as appropriate, facilitate discussion on *type* of support provided, indicate on the line with any combination of "M," "E," or "I," and add other details as needed?		
12. For each relationship, discuss the flow of resources, energy, and interest, and indicate the direction with arrows?		
Concluding the activity		
13. Discuss with the family a summary of the supports and resources and relationships with each?		
14. Ask the family what changes, if any, they would like to see in their ecomap?		
15. Discuss possible ways early intervention can help mobilize, coordinate, or provide supports to improve family satisfaction with their supports?		

CHAPTER 2

Assessing Families' Needs
with the Routines-Based Interview

R. A. McWILLIAM

When working with families with young children with special needs, one of the first orders of business is the development of the plan of how we are to help them. To make a meaningful plan, we need to assess their needs—needs for the child to acquire skills and function well and needs for the family to be able to support the child's development and learning. The Routines-Based Interview (RBI; McWilliam, 1992, 2005) is a process for the family to identify functional needs to be addressed on the individualized family service plan (IFSP; see "Brief Glossary" in the Introduction) or the individualized education program (IEP). In this chapter, I argue for the need for a functional needs assessment, followed by steps to prepare for the RBI, steps of the RBI itself, how to document results of the process, how to translate those results to IFSP outcomes or IEP goals, and a discussion of implementation challenges and solutions. As in all chapters, a checklist describing the steps of the process is provided (see Appendix 2.1), along with a checklist of elements of a quality interview (see Appendix 2.2).

THE NEED FOR A FUNCTIONAL NEEDS ASSESSMENT

First, we need functional IFSP outcomes or IEP goals because they will address (1) the child's participation in home, school (if applicable), and community routines; (2) the child's independence in those routines; and (3) the child's social relation-

27

ships in those routines. These three domains pervade a family-centered approach to early intervention in natural environments. It could be argued that many IFSPs and IEPs do not focus on these areas. Instead, they tend to be organized by relatively less functional developmental domains, such as cognitive, communication, motor, adaptive, and social–emotional.

Second, we need family priorities to be reflected in the IFSP or IEP because family input into the plan is often done in one of two ineffective ways: Either (1) families are simply asked what are their priorities and those priorities are accepted (this is what happens with many IFSPs), or (2) professionals recommend goals to families, who often just acquiesce (this is what happens with many IEPs). The problem with (1) is that, without a proper framework for families to be able to discern their priorities, they do not articulate specific functional outcomes. The problem with (2) is that family priorities are either assumed or not known. Some framework is needed to support families' identifying their priorities (see McWilliam, 2003a).

Third, outcomes or goals need to be broad yet specific enough because too many IFSPs are too broad, and too many IEPs are too narrow. By planning in the context of *function during routines*, this balance can be achieved.

Fourth, we need strategies that aim directly at the function problem. Indirect, sometimes very tangential "interventions" are often the by-product of too-general outcomes. For example, an outcome could be Peter will play with peers. Interventionists who do not understand the concept of a direct intervention might work on "underlying" problems, which they might perceive as having a "sensory" foundation or a social–emotional foundation. Therefore, instead of teaching the child to play with peers, the interventionist might give the child pressure through a weighted vest ("sensory") or engage in "affection activities." The issue is not whether these interventions are good or bad in and of themselves (see Hoehn & Baumeister, 1994), but as methods for addressing the goal of playing with peers, they are too indirect.

Fifth, caregivers other than the family need to be invested in the plan because, ultimately, we want regular caregivers providing children with learning opportunities, so they need to have some commitment to the plan. One way to get that commitment is to find out what they see as needs in those routines they share with the child. Those are functional needs. They will be addressed in program planning, which then will signal caregivers that they are listened to and counted on. Without knowing what the right cutoff is, we have used 15 hours a week as the threshold: If someone other than the parents cares for the child for 15 hours or more a week, that person is included in the needs assessment process.

Because these five points are often not addressed in traditional IFSP or IEP development and they are critical to provide a functional base for intervention, a functional needs assessment should be added to the process of receiving early intervention/early childhood special education.

The RBI is described in this chapter as a process for conducting such a functional needs assessment. It has been described elsewhere for its applicability in assessing the resource needs of families (McWilliam, 2005a), but here it is described for its broader applicability—as a method for assessing developmental and behavioral needs in the child and support needs in the family.

What Are Routines?

Routines are "everyday" activities that happen at home, in group care (e.g., child care, preschool), and the community (Bernheimer & Weisner, 2007). They might not happen literally every day, but they recur and they constitute the pattern of family and so-called school life. They are not lessons or activities imposed on natural family and school life, as in "We're going to teach the family some routines." Occasionally, we hear of families that "have no routines." By our definition, that's impossible. In all families, people wake up, are fed, change clothes, hang out, go places, and so on. Some families have little structure, which means that routines are not consistent, but the routines we inquire about are the everyday activities that happen without any interference from early intervention.

What Is the RBI?

The RBI is a semistructured interview, conducted by a professional, of at least one parent, regarding child and family functioning in daily home and school routines (Dunlap, Ester, Langhans, & Fox, 2006), for the purposes of selecting a list of functional outcomes or goals for intervention and establishing a positive relationship with the family. According to the original description of what has come to be known as the RBI, the whole process consists of five stages: preparation of families and staff, the interview itself, outcome or goal selection, outcome or goal writing, and developing strategies and reviewing progress (McWilliam, 1992).

PREPARATION FOR THE RBI

Preparing for the RBI means giving the family a number of choices and securing professionals' understanding about what will happen. Families are asked to think about their daily routines, what everyone does during them, and what changes in routines they would like to see (see Bailey et al., 1998). Professionals are similarly asked to think about routines (including classroom routines, if that's where they know the child), especially the child's engagement, independence, and social relationships in each routine (see McWilliam, 1992, for forms; see Step 5 below). Furthermore, families are asked about their preferences for who attends and where and when the meeting will take place.

STRUCTURE OF THE RBI

The RBI follows a specific structure, with some required components. These have been discovered over hundreds of applications of the RBI to be essential to a successful interview. Although derivatives of the RBI have been proposed and they serve some function, they fall short of resulting in the same benefits as the RBI. For example, many early interventionists ask about the family's typical day. The family then might recount routines, with professionals asking clarifying questions. Most often, the typical-day question is asked during intake, when first getting to know the family (see Tisot & Thurman, 2002); it is not used as the principal assessment of needs for the purpose of selecting outcomes or goals. Follow-up questions on the RBI are focused around three functional domains, and the process always ends with a list of outcomes. The framework for the RBI is found in the RBI Implementation Checklist (Appendix 2.1 at the end of this chapter). The following section describes the steps in the checklist, starting with the Interview section.

Family Interview

1. At the interview, greet the family then tell them the *purpose* for the meeting (e.g., to get to know the family and to determine how best to provide support to their child and family). It is a good idea to let them know how much time has been scheduled for the meeting and to reassure them that more time can be scheduled, if everything is not accomplished in that time.

2. Ask the parents if they have any *major questions or concerns* before starting the interview. This question is similar to the general question often asked in developing IFSPs. It tends to generate fairly general responses, which is fine in the context of the RBI but, alone, is insufficient for planning. Reassure the family that questions about their major concerns will be asked in the context of routines.

3. Ask the parents to describe their daily routines beginning with *who in the home wakes up first*. The usual question is, "How does your day start?" Asking about the parent's day signals to the family that this is not just about the child.

4. *Listen carefully* to what the parent is saying and make sure someone is taking notes. From the beginning, it is important to use verbal and nonverbal behaviors to let the family know they are being listened to (Coulehan et al., 2001). Taking notes helps convey that message.

5. Ask the parents follow-up questions to learn about the child's *engagement, independence, and social relationships*, and what other family members are doing in each routine. These are the three functional domains. Engagement is the amount of time children spend interacting with their environment in a contextually and developmentally appropriate manner, at different levels of competence (McWilliam, Scarborough, & Kim, 2003). In the context of routines, it means the quality of the child's participation in that routine, which can include the child's independence and social relationships; the three domains are not mutually exclusive. Social rela-

tionships include both communication skills and getting along with others. The interviewer asks enough questions of the family to get quite detailed information about child and family functioning in each routine.

6. At the end of the discussion about each routine, ask the family to rate their *satisfaction with the routine* on a scale from 1 (not at all satisfied) to 5 (very satisfied). One of the main purposes of early intervention should be to improve the quality of life of families of young children with disabilities (see Bailey et al., 1998). A dimension of such quality of life is the family's satisfaction with their routines. These ratings have proven useful for monitoring the effects of early intervention across repeated applications of the RBI (i.e., over time).

7. Put a star next to the notes where a family has indicated a desire for a change in routine or has said something they would like for their child or family to be able to do. Marking the potential intervention areas is necessary for the summary, so the interviewer can quickly find potential outcomes or goals. These starred items are not yet outcomes or goals; they are *concerns* that might be chosen as outcomes or goals.

8. *Avoid giving advice*. During the course of the interview, sometimes either the parent asks the professional for suggestions, or the professional itches to make suggestions. These can be masked as follow-up questions, as in, "Have you tried this?" "Have you tried that?" It is important, however, to refrain from giving advice, because that changes the dynamics of the conversation. In counseling, Egan's (1994) stage model of the skilled helper involves the stages of exploring, understanding, then action. Novice mentors are prone to jump straight to action, without acknowledging that the quality of the action (i.e., advice) depends on the quality of exploring and understanding (Garvey & Alred, 2000). While the professional makes suggestions, the parent is in the recipient, listening role. Once this stance is taken, families are sometimes more reluctant to discuss what happens in routines without checking in with the professional ("Is that right? Is that what I should be doing?"). If the family directly asks for advice, the professional should acknowledge it is a great question and promise to have it answered later. Then, it is important to come back to it, after the interview.

9. Ask the family, "When you lie awake at night, worrying, what is it you *worry* about?" The worry question was used in a series of case studies about service utilization (Harbin, McWilliam, & Gallagher, 2000) and proved to provide such important information that it has been incorporated into the RBI for those professionals comfortable asking it. This question and the next one can provoke emotion in the family, so they should be handled sensitively. Sometimes, families will say they spend no time lying awake because they are dead tired, but then they should simply be asked if there's anything they worry about. Some follow-up questions or comments must be made to show interest and empathy. For example, the most common answer to this question is something about money, so a reasonable follow-up question might be, "Have you run into any problems yet or are you worried that you won't have enough money for things in the future?" A reasonable

comment might be, "It's hard when you don't know what your child will need, isn't it?"

10. Ask the family, "If you could *change* anything about your life, what would it be?" The change question is a variation on the miracle question, which is common in solution-focused brief therapy (Popescu, 2005). The miracle question in counseling is something akin to "If a miracle were to occur relative to the problem that brought you to therapy, what would your life look like?" In working with families of children with disabilities, we do not ask the question that way, because if their answer is that their child would not have a disability, there is nothing much we can do with that. Rewording it as a change question allows the family to focus on what is manageable.

11. Ask the family if there is *anything else* that should be added to their list of concerns. Because not everything happens in routines, it is helpful to check in with the family about other concerns. Most often, families have nothing to add, because the conversation about routines elicits information about both the routines themselves and much more.

Teacher Interview

Teachers are interviewed only if the child is in group care (i.e., being cared for with other children) for about 15 hours a week or more. "Teachers" are any caregivers in group care such as child care or preschool.

12. Conduct the interview either immediately *following the family interview* or before the RBI with the family (i.e., not after the RBI). Ideally, the family and the teacher get to hear each other's report of routines. The family should go first, so they understand that their perspectives are the most important and so they do not feel they need to match the teacher. If it cannot be arranged for both to be present at the same time, the teacher should be interviewed earlier. Otherwise, three visits (family, teacher, family) instead of two (teacher, family) would be necessary, because the parents are the ones choosing the outcomes. At the second visit, the interviewer then conveys what the teacher has reported.

13. If the teacher interview was done earlier, the interviewer reports to the parent the teacher's information *routine by routine*. Although special education and related-service professionals are used to reporting on children's abilities by developmental domain (e.g., cognitive, communication, motor, adaptive, social), a more meaningful categorization is by routine. Families and teachers can picture the child in everyday situations, events, and activities, whereas developmental domains—think of "cognitive," for example—are harder to see in one's mind's eye. Therefore, child functioning is not reported by domain by going through all of a child's cognitive skills, communication, motor, and so on. Discussing routines keeps the conversation more functional.

14. Ask the teacher to describe each of the *classroom routines* from the time of the child's arrival through departure. Classroom routines are usually dictated by the classroom schedule. Infant care has less structure, but, starting with toddler care, classrooms will have schedules.

15. *Listen carefully* to what the teacher is saying and make sure someone is taking notes. As with interviewing families, it is important to interview teachers in a way that encourages them to provide much information.

16. Ask the teacher *follow-up questions* to learn about the child's engagement, independence, and social competence, and what other children are doing in each routine. The functional domains keep the focus on child functioning and not on test-based domains or on disciplines such as physical therapy, occupational therapy, or speech therapy. The information about what the other children are doing allows the interviewer and family to know what the expectations or group norms are for that routine.

17. At the end of each routine, ask the teacher to rate the *goodness of fit* between the routine and the child. Note that, unlike with home routines the teacher's satisfaction with the routine is not the most important issue. For example, a teacher might be highly satisfied with a routine that permitted no creativity but that resulted in no conflict. More important than the teacher's satisfaction is whether the routine is working for this individual child. The concept of goodness of fit allows the evaluation not to be about deficits in the child or weaknesses in the activities, but rather about the match between the child and the specific routine.

18. Put a *star* next to the notes where the teacher has indicated a desire for a change in routine or has said something that he or she would like the child to be able to do. Again, it is important to mark areas requiring further information or concerns the teacher has illustrated, so the interviewer can review them quickly in Step 20.

19. Ask the teacher if there is *anything else* that should be added to the list of classroom concerns. Occasionally, teachers will have concerns beyond what is discussed in routines.[1]

20. *Review all home and classroom concerns* (starred) with the parents. The purpose of the review is simply to remind the family of potential outcomes. This review should be done quite quickly.

---

[1] A frequently asked question is, "What do you do when a family comes up with a completely unrealistic outcome or goal?" which usually means one that is too advanced for the child. Our typical response to this scenario is to affirm the family's goal (i.e., "That's a really good thing to work toward") and to ask them what they think we should work on as a first step toward achieving that goal. If, for example, a family says they want the child to tell about their day, and the child currently is only babbling (i.e., no words), the interviewer should say, "That's a great goal. Considering right now she's still just babbling, what do you think she'll be able to do next?" If necessary, the interviewer can suggest that real words might be the next skill. The point is to affirm the family's goal and help them identify a way to get there.

21. Ask the family to *list the things* they would like the team *to work on*. Prompt the family as necessary. A symbolic and somewhat dramatic gesture here can be to hand over all the notes (or the RBI Report Form [Appendix 2.2], if that was used to record information) to the family, so they can see the starred items. Handing over notes shows the family the interviewer has nothing to hide and that they are partners. Note that the family, not professionals, is selecting outcomes. The interviewer might or might not retrieve the notes. They are not kept as an official document.

22. Ask the family what goal they would most like to have help with (i.e., first priority goal or outcome). Ask the family what their next priority is and continue *prioritizing goals* until all of the concerns the family wants on the plan are included. This step can produce surprising priorities, although what is predictable is that many families put family-level outcomes or goals at the end. Prioritizing goals becomes important during intervention because it can be difficult to attend to all outcomes or goals equally.

23. *If time permits*, once all of the goals are chosen by the parent, specialists share information about how goals might be addressed (i.e., *strategy planning*). This could happen at another meeting. In some communities, "strategies" are required before the IFSP is finished. Many IFSP forms have space for strategies for each outcome, and states vary in their guidance about what should go in that space. Generally, strategies are the procedures the team will use to address the outcome, such as "full physical prompt" or "at least four play times a day." One or two general strategies are the most that can be expected at this stage of intervention planning. With new children, the IFSP or IEP development process happens too fast for the kind of functional assessment that would lead to specific strategies. Such strategies should be added to the IFSP as they are developed.

24. Discuss with the team *when services will be decided upon*—at this meeting or a subsequent one. This is a vital part of the IFSP, although not as vital as the outcome selection process, because services are based on outcomes, not vice versa.

25. *Thank everyone* for their time. Compliment the family on what a good, functional list of outcomes they decided upon. Indeed, if the RBI went well, the list will be a good one.

These 25 steps describe a process for assessing functional needs after eligibility has been determined. The list of outcomes or goals is the basis for completing the IFSP or IEP.

Keys to a Successful Interview

The first key to a successful interview is to follow the RBI Report Form (Appendix 2.2) or at least to stick to the structure shown in the interview. As mentioned earlier, shortcuts inevitably result in less-than-satisfactory information and too few outcomes or goals.

The quality of the interview hinges largely on the quality of the follow-up questions, which cannot be defined; they are idiosyncratic to the family and, to some extent, the interests and background of the interviewer(s). Many follow-up questions are closed-ended questions to find out how the child participates in the routine (i.e., is engaged): "Does he do this? Does she do that?" The interviewer has to know enough about child development and family functioning to make these questions relevant. The evaluative questions about satisfaction with the routine or the goodness of fit between the routine and the child are powerful. Rating families' and teachers' perceptions appears to be an improvement over simply asking the questions.

Various nonverbal behaviors are important. It is helpful to sit at right angles with the person answering most of the questions. This allows the parent to see what the interviewer is writing and to make eye contact but also to look away. The primary interviewer should keep the paper down, so the family can see if they choose to.

A few other hints are as follows:

- Relax; don't ask a checklist of questions.
- Show real interest; don't make it look perfunctory.
- Empathize; don't be poker-faced.
- Accept; don't judge. This is probably the most important hint.
- Use your strengths; don't assume everyone's style is the same. That means use humor if you're funny; be touchy-feely if you're touchy-feely. Be genuine. People who naturally are formal might have some challenges, because an informal, friendly approach has been so successful.

Key Statements and Questions

The structure of the RBI has been provided earlier in this chapter, but the following key statements and questions might be a reminder.

- *"You don't have to answer any questions you don't want to."* This reassurance is necessary because we are asking about private family lives. It is the first thing we say. Most families appear to be very open.
- *"Who is in your family?"* If this information has not been gathered earlier, it is necessary, because in each routine the functions of everyone in the family are asked about.
- *"Briefly describe your child."* Variations on this request are the way to get a sense of what the child's disabilities are. The interviewer will often have this information from prior paperwork, but it is still useful to hear how the family describes the child.
- *"What are your main concerns?"* This question is the equivalent of the ineffectual open question traditionally used to determine IFSP outcomes—the question

that results in two or three lame outcomes. It is, however, important to find out what families are most concerned about when they begin the meeting. Sometimes the final outcomes reflect these concerns. Sometimes they don't.

• *"How does your day begin?"* Asking the parents how their day begins shows that this is about all family members, not just the "client" child.

• *For each routine, get the six pieces of critical information.* They are (1) what everyone else is doing, (2) what this child is doing, (3) what the child's engagement or participation in the routine is like, (4) what his or her independence in the routine is like, (5) what his or her social relationships in the routine are like, and (6) how satisfactory the routine is or how well it fits with the child.

• *"What happens after that?"* Transitions in the conversation from routine to routine should be handled to allow the family to paint the picture, rather than asking about specific routines.

• *"Let's skip to _____."* If the interview is taking up too much time, the interviewer might ask to skip to routines presumably happening later in the day.

• *"Let me remind you of the concerns you mentioned."* Once routines have been described and the worry and change questions asked (see p. 31–32), the interviewer looks back through the notes and mentions the concerns he or she had starred.

• *"What would you like the team to work on?"* This is the development of the outcomes or goals list. The interviewer writes down fairly shorthand versions, often incorporating the family's language.

• *If necessary, remind the parent of issues that arose during the interview.* Handing the family the notes with starred items is helpful.

• *"Which is the most important of these? And then?"* Asking families to put the plan into priority order ends the outcome selection process.

DOCUMENTING RESULTS

The RBI was originally developed with no additional paperwork burden. Curiously, as much as early interventionists hate paperwork, without it they are often lost. The RBI Report Form (McWilliam, 2003b) was developed to provide guidance about what to ask about in routines. The latest version, unveiled here, retains the original format but adds an outcome or goal page and incorporates prompt questions.

The RBI Report Form

Directions for using the RBI Report Form are provided on the form itself. The directions state that two versions of the routines pages exist: (1) an "open" form that does not specify the routine being discussed or specific questions to ask about, and (2) a "structured" form, on which home routines and exact questions are specified (see Appendix 2.3, RBI–SAFER Combo). This structured form is a combination of the original RBI Report Form and the Scale for Assessment of Family Enjoyment within Routines (SAFER; Scott & McWilliam, 2000). The RBI Report Form is printed with one open routines page, so more copies of that page are needed. Programs and families can decide whether the completed forms are considered official paperwork that others would have access to or are simply tools to help the interviewer complete the interview.

Examples of Informal Outcomes from RBIs

The following lists are real outcomes derived from an RBI. They are listed exactly as written by the interviewer, based on what the interviewed parents said. They would subsequently be restated to be measurable, as discussed in the next section.

Julia's Priorities

1. Nicholas communicates his needs (drink, don't feel well, eat, "more," play, TV, outside)
2. Eating with combination of textures; vegetables, fruits
3. Handwashing—water rinsing
4. Identifying objects (in a book, on body), to see where Nicholas is cognitively
5. Transitions (e.g., from park) when Nicholas has to stop doing something fun
6. Therapies more under Julia's control
7. Child care when Julia needs longer-term care (e.g., during her medical treatments)

Karen's Outcomes

1. Making sounds (playing with David, diaper, reading, play, feeding)
2. Responding to Emily and David during reading, play, meals
3. Reach (playing on floor, bath, swim class, music, feeding)
4. Batting for toys and splashing (play, bath)
5. Grasp things in front of him (music, bath, feeding)
6. Rolling both ways, pushing up (play)
7. Sitting unassisted (music, bath, feeding)
8. Information on research, what other moms do, bedtime rituals
9. Time for David and Emily together (get parents here)

Melanie's Outcomes for Eric

1. No more biting
2. Use words and other alternatives to actions to get what he wants (leaving, transitions at school, other activities)

3. Focus on activity longer (snack/lunch, story, teacher-led activities, free play, table-top)
4. Information about toe turning in and other medical resources
5. Make transitions more smoothly
6. Using spoon without turning over (breakfast and other meals)
7. Help with undressing (bath time)
8. Change housing to place with land and safe neighborhood

From RBI to IFSP Outcomes or IEP Goals

When conducted according to the guidelines presented here, the RBI produces very functional outcomes, ideal for an IFSP or IEP, but for the fact that they would need to be reworded to meet accountability criteria. Some early interventionists believe the addition of criteria ruins family-friendly outcomes. On the other hand, it might be condescending to think that families would not care about what exactly is being targeted and when it has been accomplished. It is beyond the scope of this chapter to provided detailed guidance about functional outcome or goal writing. The following seven steps have, however, been adopted in a number of communities, following our training.

Steps to Writing a Functional Child Outcome

A functional outcome must, by definition, come from a functional assessment. One cannot take a nonfunctional "goal" and turn it into a functional one by writing it well; you will simply end up with a well-written nonfunctional outcome. A functional, family-centered assessment of needs is critical for writing a functional outcome.

1. *Read the shorthand version of the outcome* from a family-centered, functional needs assessment (e.g., RBI). The result of such an assessment would be a list of priorities the family has chosen. The interviewer writes down the outcome, initially, without consideration of the exact wording to be used on the IFSP. An example from an RBI in which the parents described a child who ate only pureed foods was "chewing food."

2. *Find out what routines this affects.* Having done an RBI, one would of course know this. In the example above, the parents wanted their child, Darcy, to be able to handle solid foods at lunch, at dinner, and in restaurants. They were not worried about breakfast, when they were in a hurry: They were content to let Darcy eat pureed foods at that time.

3. *Write "[Child] will participate in [the routine(s) in question]."* This idea, which came from Pip Campbell, an eminent occupational therapist, educator, and researcher at Thomas Jefferson University in Philadelphia, emphasizes engagement in routines. Almost every child-level outcome can be worded this way if a

routines-based assessment was conducted. In the example given, then, we would write, "Darcy will participate in breakfast, in lunch, and in restaurants." Make sure it is worded in terms of routines in which the child will participate, not replacing the routine with a behavior class. For example, if the priority was that Allan will play with his sister, and the routines in which this need arose were waiting for breakfast and waiting for dinner, we would not write, "Allan will participate in play with his sister." We would, instead, write, "Allan will participate in playtime before breakfast and dinner."

4. *Write "by _____ing," addressing the specific behaviors.* This is where the specific behavior is identified, so, in our example, it could read, "by chewing food and swallowing it."

5. *Add a criterion for demonstrating that the child has acquired the skill.* A handy way to think about the acquisition criterion is to think and possibly write, "We will know she can do this when. . . . " This is the first measurable criterion. How would we know when Darcy could chew and swallow? Should we count the number of chews?: too difficult to see and too variable, depending on the type and amount of food in her mouth. The team decided to let the parents decide on whether the chewing (and swallowing) was occurring but to propose a volume criterion. They suggested 1 cup, which the parents thought was reasonable: If Darcy could eat 1 cup of food in this manner, we would know she could indeed chew food and swallow it. So the criterion was written as "We will know she can do this when she eats 1 cup of food in this manner."

6. *Add another criterion for generalization, maintenance, or fluency, if appropriate.* Do we simply want Darcy to chew and swallow 1 cup of food, some time, somewhere, and then we're done? No. A generalization-across-routines criterion is built into the outcome already: We want her to be able to eat 1 cup of food in this manner at lunch, at dinner, and at a restaurant. The nature of routines-based assessments such as the RBI is that generalization across routines will often be this second criterion. Generalization can also be programmed across people, materials, places, and so on (Stokes & Baer, 1977). Instead of a generalization criterion, it might be more appropriate to have a criterion for the rate of behavior, which is fluency. For example, if a child can walk but the parent wants her to walk faster, a criterion might be that she walks 10 paces in 20 seconds. A maintenance criterion is warranted when the parent is concerned that the child will stop performing a skill he or she has learned.

7. *Over what amount of time?* As currently written, it might be possible for Darcy to chew and swallow 1 cup of food at lunch in December, 1 cup of food at dinner in January, and 1 cup of food in a restaurant in February. Is that what was meant? No, to be convinced that Darcy could chew and swallow, we would need to see if she could do so in each of those places in 1 week. Note that the exact measurement criteria are proposals; there is nothing magical about them. If one knows the baseline amount (i.e., what the child is already doing at the time of the assessment), it helps to set reasonable criteria. Otherwise, we are simply establishing a target, on the

principle that having realistic goals is associated with good performance (Earley & Lituchy, 1991). The whole outcome, then, reads as follows: "Darcy will participate in breakfast, in lunch, and in restaurants, by chewing and swallowing her food. We will know she can do this when she eats 1 cup of food in this manner, one time at lunch, one time at dinner, and one time in a restaurant, in 1 week."

Some professionals are concerned, on first hearing about the RBI, that they will have difficulty establishing measurable outcomes. As can be seen here, the general outcome of chewing and swallowing became (1) highly measurable and (2) functional by virtue of the emphasis on participation in specific routines.

Family-Level Outcomes

Family-level outcomes do not need to be so heavily measurable, but they should still be measurable to some extent. Usually, we develop one criterion. Unlike child-level outcomes that involve some editing of the wording, family-level outcomes should usually remain close to the family's actual words. Table 2.1 shows the conversion from the shorthand to the IFSP wording.

The field has not developed family-level goals as originally envisioned when Public Law 99-142 was passed (Garwood, 1987). The IEP mentality has possibly been responsible for this failure. This mentality includes the belief that the system is responsible for ensuring that any goal on the plan is met, which might mean applying resources (e.g., services) to get the goal met (Turnbull et al., 2007). The IFSP mentality, however, should not follow that line of thinking. On the IFSP, the "measurable results or outcomes expected to be achieved for the infant or toddler and the family" [Individuals with Disabilities Education Improvement Act; IDEIA, 2004, Public Law 108-446, Part C, Sec. 636 (d) (3)] should be written. Nowhere in the law does it state that there should be a one-to-one correspondence between outcomes and services, even though some states organize their IFSP forms that way. Instead, the IFSP must contain "a statement of specific early intervention services . . . necessary to meet the unique needs of the infant or toddler and the

TABLE 2.1. Conversion from Shorthand to IFSP Wording

Shorthand wording	IFSP wording
Alicia more time for herself	Alicia will have 2 hours to herself, without child care responsibilities, every 2 weeks for 3 months.
Don and Karen go out	Don and Karen will go out together, without Cameron, once by June and once again by September.
Safe housing	The Morellis will have information about three affordable options for safe housing.
Van big enough for travel chair	Hilda will buy a van big enough for Ricky's travel chair by June.
Mary get a job	Mary will be employed for at least 20 hours a week by November.

family." Service coordination or any of the other early intervention services can support the family in meeting their "unique needs" (McWilliam, 2006; Roberts, 2006). Such support can be through providing information. We are not required to babysit children while parents have time for themselves or go out together, to provide safe housing, to buy vehicles, or to employ parents. But we can give parents emotional support and information about financial and other resources to address their family-level needs.

IMPLEMENTATION CHALLENGES AND SOLUTIONS

To implement the RBI, communities will need to decide when in the IFSP or IEP development it should be conducted (see McWilliam, 2005a). Options might be at intake, evaluation, between evaluation and the IFSP or IEP meeting, or during the IFSP or IEP meeting. Most communities choose the third option, although increasingly programs are choosing the second option, by scoring instruments primarily from families' reports during the RBI.

If more than 10% of the children tested for eligibility are proven to be ineligible, programs should consider a screening or conducting eligibility determination before the RBI. Otherwise, it is expensive to conduct an RBI on an ineligible child, and it can mislead the family.

The meeting itself can have different combinations of people in attendance, but the family should decide on the group's constitution. The child does not have to be present for the RBI. Families should be told that it is helpful to everyone to have interruptions minimized but they should not feel guilty if they cannot alter the environment. From the point of view of the interviewers, it is helpful to have two interviewers, although one is manageable. If two are used, the second one's role can be to help by asking additional questions, taking notes, handling interruptions, and, possibly, scoring a developmental test.

CONCLUSION

In conclusion, the RBI is a powerful tool that early interventionists and early childhood special education teachers and their administrators can use to plan functional intervention plans and to establish positive relationships with families. Although a primary service provider approach is not necessary for using the RBI, this planning strategy does establish a philosophical base for a transdisciplinary model. This base contains the principles that children learn all the time from their natural caregivers, so services should be designed to support caregivers for times between visits or sessions. The RBI produces a wealth of information about child and family functioning that makes intervention planning (i.e., strategies) easy. The information helps professionals figure out potential strategies, and families learn the strategies as they go through the prioritized, functional outcomes between visits. The contacts themselves are for the exchange of information, for encouragement to the family, and for attention to all family members. But it all begins with a functional intervention plan derived from the RBI.

REFERENCES

Bailey, D. B., McWilliam, R. A., Darkes, L. A., Hebbler, K., Simeonsson, R. J., Spiker, D., et al. (1998). Family outcomes in early intervention: A framework for program evaluation and efficacy research. *Exceptional Children, 64,* 313–328.

Bernheimer, L. P., & Weisner, T. S. (2007). "Let me just tell you what I do all day. . . . ": The family story at the center of intervention research and practice. *Infants and Young Children, 20*(3), 192–201.

Coulehan, J. L., Platt, F. W., Egener, B., Frankel, R., Lin, C., Lown, B., et al. (2001). "Let me see if I have this right. . . . ": Words that help build empathy. *Annals of Internal Medicine, 135,* 221–227.

Dunlap, G., Ester, T., Langhans, S., & Fox, L. (2006). Functional communication training with toddlers in home environments. *Journal of Early Intervention, 28*(2), 81–96.

Earley, P. C., & Lituchy, T. R. (1991). Delineating goal and efficacy effects: A test of three models. *Journal of Applied Psychology, 76*(1), 81.

Egan, G. (1994). *The skilled helper: A problem-management approach to helping* (4th ed.). Pacific Grove, CA: Brookes/Cole.

Garvey, B., & Alred, G. (2000). Developing mentors. *Career Development International, 5/4/5,* 216–222.

Garwood, S. G. (1987). Politics, economics, and practical issues affecting the development of universal early intervention for handicapped infants. *Topics in Early Childhood Special Education, 7*(2), 6–18.

Harbin, G. L., McWilliam, R. A., & Gallagher, J. J. (2000). Services for young children with disabilities and their families. In J. P. Shonkoff & S. J. Meisels (Eds.), *Handbook of early intervention* (2nd ed., pp. 387–415). Cambridge, UK: Cambridge University Press.

Hoehn, T. P., & Baumeister, A. A. (1994). A critique of the application of sensory integration therapy to children with learning disabilities. *Journal of Learning Disabilities, 27,* 338–350.

Individuals with Disabilities Education Improvement Act. (2004). Public Law 108-446, Part C, Sec. 636 (d)(3).

McWilliam, R. A. (1992). *Family-centered intervention planning: A routines-based approach.* Tucson, AZ: Communication Skill Builders.

McWilliam, R. A. (2003a). Giving families a chance to talk so they can plan. *News Exchange, 8*(3), 1, 4–6.

McWilliam, R. A. (2003b). *RBI report form.* Nashville, TN: Vanderbilt University Medical Center.

McWilliam, R. A. (2005). Assessing the resource needs of families in the context of early intervention. In M. J. Guralnick (Ed.), *A developmental systems approach to early intervention* (pp. 215–234). Baltimore: Brookes.

McWilliam, R. A. (2006). What happened to service coordination? *Journal of Early Intervention, 28*(3), 166–168.

McWilliam, R. A., Scarborough, A. A., & Kim, H. (2003). Adult interactions and child engagement. *Early Education and Development, 14,* 7–27.

Popescu, B. (2005). Paradigm shift in the therapeutic approach: An overview of solution-focused brief therapy. *Europe's Journal of Psychology,* February. Retrieved from *www.ejop.org/archives/2005/02/paradigm_shift.html.*

Roberts, R. N. (2006). Wow! Models of service coordination do make a difference. *Journal of Early Intervention, 28*(3), 169–171.

Scott, S., & McWilliam, R. A. (2000). *Scale for assessment of family enjoyment within routines (SAFER).* FPG Child Development Institute, University of North Carolina at Chapel Hill (available at www.siskin.org).

Stokes, T. F., & Baer, D. M. (1977). An implicit technology of generalization. *Journal of Applied Behavior Analysis, 10*(2), 349–367.

Tisot, C. M., & Thurman, S. K. (2002). Using behavior setting theory to define natural settings: A family-centered approach. *Infants and Young Children, 14*(3), 65–71.

Turnbull, A. P., Summers, A. J., Turnbull, R., Brotherson, M. J., Winton, P., Roberts, R., et al. (2007). Family supports and services in early intervention: A bold vision. *Journal of Early Intervention, 29*(3), 187–206.

RBI Implementation Checklist

Interviewer _____ Date _____

Observer _____ Score _____

	+	±	–	Comments
1. Did the interviewer prepare the family, at least the day before the interview, by telling them (a) that they will be asked to describe their daily routines, (b) they can choose a location, and (c) they can choose who participates (including whether it's one or both parents)?				
2. Did the interviewer greet the family and then review the purpose for the meeting (e.g., to get to know the family and to determine how best to provide support to their child and family)?				
3. Did the interviewer ask the parents whether they have any major questions or concerns before starting the interview?				
4. Did the interview have a good flow (i.e., conversational, not a lot of time spent writing)?				
5. Did the interviewer maintain focus without attending too much to distractions?				
6. Did the interviewer ask follow-up questions to gain an understanding of functioning?				
7. Did the interviewer address all of the family's routines, especially by following the parent's lead?				

Goal 85% or better (total score of 87 or better on numbered items)
Scoring: +3 points +/– 2 points – 0 points

(cont.)

	+	±	−	Comments
8. Were there follow-up questions related to engagement?				
9. Were there follow-up questions related to independence?				
10. Were there follow-up questions related to social relationships?				
11. Were follow-up questions developmentally appropriate?				
12. Were open-ended questions used initially to gain an understanding of the routine and functioning (followed by closed-ended questions if necessary)?				
13. Did the interviewer find out what people in the family other than the child are doing in each routine?				
14. Did the interviewer ask for a rating of each routine?				
15. Did the interviewer find out how satisfied the family is with each routine through both description and rating?				
16. To transition between routines, was the question "What happens next?" or something similar used?				
17. Did the interviewer use good affect (e.g. facial expressions, tone of voice, responsiveness)?				
18. Did the interviewer use affirming behaviors (e.g., nodding, positive comments, or gestures)?				

(cont.)

	+	±	–	Comments
19. Did the interviewer attempt to get the parent's perspective on behaviors (why he or she thinks the child does what he or she does)?				
20. Did the interviewer use active listening techniques (e.g., rephrasing, clarifying, summarizing)?				
21. If there were no problems in the routine, did the interviewer ask what the parent would next like to see?				
22. Did the interviewer avoid giving advice?				
23. Did the interviewer avoid unnecessary questions, such as the specific time something occurs?				
24. Did the interviewer act in a nonjudgmental way?				
25. Did the interviewer use "time of day" instead of "routine"?				
26. Did the interviewer return easily to the interview after an interruption?				
27. Did the interviewer allow the family to state their own opinions, concerns, and so on (not leading the family toward what the interviewer thinks is important)?				
28. Did the interviewer get information on the parent's downtime (any time for him- or herself)?				

(cont.)

	+	±	–	Comments
29. Ask the family, "When you lie awake at night worrying, what is it you worry about?"				
30. Ask the family, "If you could change anything about your life, what would it be?"				
31. Did the interviewer put a star next to the notes where a family has indicated a desire for change in routine or has said something they would like for their child or family to be able to do?				
32. After the interviewer has summarized concerns, was the family asked whether anything should be added?				
33. After summarizing concerns (starred items), did the interviewer take out a clean sheet of paper and ask the family what they wanted to work on? (New List)				
34. Did the interviewer ask the family to put the outcomes into a priority order for importance?				
35. Did the interviewer discuss when the services will be decided upon—at this meeting or a subsequent one?				
36. Did the interviewer thank everyone for their time?				

RBI Report Form

Directions:

This form is designed to be used to report the findings from the McWilliam model of conducting a routines-based interview. A second person (e.g., someone assisting the lead interviewer) can use the form to summarize the discussion during the interview, or it can be filled out at the end of the interview. Two versions of the routines pages exist: (1) an "open" form that does not specify the routine being discussed or specific questions to ask about, and (2) a "structured" form, on which home routines and exact questions are specified. This structured form is a combination of the original RBI Report Form and the Scale for Assessment of Family Enjoyment within Routines (SAFER; Scott & McWilliam, 2000).

1. Complete the information below.
2. For each routine, write a short phrase defining the routine (e.g., *waking up, breakfast, hanging out, circle, snack, centers*).
3. Write brief descriptions about the child's engagement in the "Engagement" box (e.g., *Participates with breakfast routine, banging spoon on the high chair* or *Pays attention to the teacher; names songs when asked; often leaves circle before it has ended*).
4. If the interview revealed no information about one of the three domains, circle "No information" in that domain for that routine.
5. Write brief descriptions about the child's independence in the "Independence" box (e.g., *Feeds herself with a spoon; drinks from a cup but spills a lot* or *Sings all the songs with the group, but needs prompting to speak loudly enough*).
6. Write brief descriptions about the child's communication and social competence in the "Social Relationships" box (e.g., *Looks parent in the eye when pointing to things in the kitchen* or *Pays attention to the teacher at circle but can't stand touching other children*).

Child's name	
Date of birth	
Who is being interviewed	
Interviewer	
Date of interview	
"What are your main concerns?"	

Make extra copies of page 2!

(cont.)

Routine	
Engagement	No information
Independence	No information
Social relationships	No information

Home: Satisfaction with routine (CIRCLE ONE) 1. Not at all satisfied 2. 3. Satisfied 4. 5. Very satisfied	*Classroom*: Fit of routine and child (CIRCLE ONE) 1. Poor goodness of fit 2. 3. Average goodness of fit 4. 5. Excellent goodness of fit

Domains addressed (CIRCLE ALL THAT APPLY):

Physical   Cognitive   Communication   Social or emotional   Adaptive

(cont.)

Outcomes

Before asking the family to select "things to work on," review the concerns identified (i.e., starred) on the previous pages.

Outcome (short, informal version)	Priority number

RBI–SAFER Combo

Routine:	Waking up

- Could you describe what wake-up time is like?
- Who usually wakes up first?
- Where does your child sleep?
- How does your child let you know she is awake?
- Does she want to be picked up right away? If so, is she happy when picked up?
- Or is she content by herself for a few minutes? What does she do?
- What is the rest of the family doing at this time?
- Is this a good time of day? If not, what would you like to be different?

Notes	
Engagement	No information
Independence	No information
Social Relationships	No information

Home: Satisfaction with routine (CIRCLE ONE)	*Classroom*: Fit of routine and child (CIRCLE ONE)
1. Not at all satisfied	1. Poor goodness of fit
2.	2.
3. Satisfied	3. Average goodness of fit
4.	4.
5. Very satisfied	5. Excellent goodness of fit

Domains addressed (CIRCLE ALL THAT APPLY):

Physical   Cognitive   Communication   Social or emotional   Adaptive

(cont.)

Combination of the Routines-Based Interview Report Form (McWilliam, 2003b) and the Scale for Assessment of Family Enjoyment within Routines (Scott & McWilliam, 2000).

Routine:	Diapering/Dressing

- What about dressing? How does that go?
- Who helps your child dress?
- Does he help with dressing? How? What can he do on his own?
- What is his mood like?
- What is communication like?
- Does your child wear diapers?
- Are there any problems with diapering?
- What does your child do while you are changing him?
- Does your child use the toilet? How independently?
- How does he let you know when he needs to use the toilet?
- How satisfied are you with this routine? Is there anything you would like to be different?

Notes	
Engagement	No information
Independence	No information
Social relationships	No information

Home: Satisfaction with routine (CIRCLE ONE)	*Classroom*: Fit of routine and child (CIRCLE ONE)
1. Not at all satisfied	1. Poor goodness of fit
2.	2.
3. Satisfied	3. Average goodness of fit
4.	4.
5. Very satisfied	5. Excellent goodness of fit

Domains addressed (CIRCLE ALL THAT APPLY):

Physical   Cognitive   Communication   Social or emotional   Adaptive

(cont.)

Routine:	Feeding/Meals

- What are feedings/mealtimes like?
- Does anyone help feed your child? Who?
- How often does she eat?
- How much can she do on her own?
- How involved is she with meals?
- Where does your child usually eat?
- What are other family members doing at this time?
- How does your child let you know what she wants or whether she is finished?
- Does she like mealtimes? How do you know?
- What would make mealtimes more enjoyable for you?
- What are mealtimes like for your child when under the care of others?

Notes	
Engagement	No information
Independence	No information
Social relationships	No information

Home: Satisfaction with routine (CIRCLE ONE)	**Classroom**: Fit of routine and child (CIRCLE ONE)
1. Not at all satisfied	1. Poor goodness of fit
2.	2.
3. Satisfied	3. Average goodness of fit
4.	4.
5. Very satisfied	5. Excellent goodness of fit

Domains addressed (CIRCLE ALL THAT APPLY):

Physical   Cognitive   Communication   Social or emotional   Adaptive

(cont.)

Routine:	Getting ready to go/traveling

- How do things go when you are getting ready to go somewhere with your child?
- Who usually helps your child get ready?
- How much can he do on his own?
- How involved is he in the whole process of getting ready to go?
- What is communication like at this time?
- Does your child like outings? How do you know?
- Is this a stressful activity? What would make this time easier for you?
- What are drop-off and pick-up times like for your child? Do you or other caregivers have any concerns?

Notes	
Engagement	No information
Independence	No information
Social relationships	No information

Home: Satisfaction with routine (CIRCLE ONE)	*Classroom*: Fit of routine and child (CIRCLE ONE)
1. Not at all satisfied	1. Poor goodness of fit
2.	2.
3. Satisfied	3. Average goodness of fit
4.	4.
5. Very satisfied	5. Excellent goodness of fit

Domains addressed (CIRCLE ALL THAT APPLY):

Physical   Cognitive   Communication   Social or emotional   Adaptive

(cont.)

Routine:	Hanging out/watching TV

- What does your family do when relaxing at home?
- How is your child involved in this activity?
- How does your child interact with other family members?
- Does your family watch TV? Will your child watch TV?
- What does he like to watch? How long will he watch TV?
- Do you have a favorite show?
- Is there anything you would like to do in the evening but can't?

Notes	
Engagement	No information
Independence	No information
Social relationships	No information

Home: Satisfaction with routine (CIRCLE ONE)	*Classroom*: Fit of routine and child (CIRCLE ONE)
1. Not at all satisfied	1. Poor goodness of fit
2.	2.
3. Satisfied	3. Average goodness of fit
4.	4.
5. Very satisfied	5. Excellent goodness of fit

Domains addressed (CIRCLE ALL THAT APPLY):

Physical   Cognitive   Communication   Social or emotional   Adaptive

(cont.)

Routine:	Bath time

- What is bath time like?
- Who usually helps your child bathe?
- How is she positioned in the bathtub?
- Does she like the water? How do you know?
- How involved is your child in bathing herself or playing in the water?
- Does she kick or splash in the water?
- What toys does she like to play with in the tub?
- How does she communicate with you? What do you talk about?
- Is bath time usually a good time? If not, what would make it better?

Notes	
Engagement	No information
Independence	No information
Social relationships	No information

Home: Satisfaction with routine (CIRCLE ONE)	*Classroom*: Fit of routine and child (CIRCLE ONE)
1. Not at all satisfied	1. Poor goodness of fit
2.	2.
3. Satisfied	3. Average goodness of fit
4.	4.
5. Very satisfied	5. Excellent goodness of fit

Domains addressed (CIRCLE ALL THAT APPLY):

Physical   Cognitive   Communication   Social or emotional   Adaptive

(cont.)

Routine:	Nap/bedtime

- How does bedtime go?
- Who usually puts your child to bed?
- Do you read books or have some type of ritual at this time?
- How does he fall asleep?
- How does your child calm himself?
- Does he sleep through the night? What happens if he wakes up? Who gets up with him?
- Is bedtime an easy or stressful time for your family?
- Does he take naps for other caregivers? How does that go?

Notes	
Engagement	No information
Independence	No information
Social relationships	No information

Home: Satisfaction with routine (CIRCLE ONE)	*Classroom*: Fit of routine and child (CIRCLE ONE)
1. Not at all satisfied	1. Poor goodness of fit
2.	2.
3. Satisfied	3. Average goodness of fit
4.	4.
5. Very satisfied	5. Excellent goodness of fit

Domains addressed (CIRCLE ALL THAT APPLY):

Physical   Cognitive   Communication   Social or emotional   Adaptive

(cont.)

Routine:	Grocery store

- How are trips to the grocery? Do you bring your child with you?
- Does she sit in a shopping cart?
- Does she like being at the store?
- How is she involved in shopping? Do you have to occupy her or is she pretty content?
- How does she react to other people in the store?
- How does she communicate with you and others at this time?
- Is there anything that would make shopping with your child easier?

Notes	
Engagement	No information
Independence	No information
Social relationships	No information

Home: Satisfaction with routine (CIRCLE ONE)	*Classroom*: Fit of routine and child (CIRCLE ONE)
1. Not at all satisfied	1. Poor goodness of fit
2.	2.
3. Satisfied	3. Average goodness of fit
4.	4.
5. Very satisfied	5. Excellent goodness of fit

Domains addressed (CIRCLE ALL THAT APPLY):

Physical   Cognitive   Communication   Social or emotional   Adaptive

(cont.)

Routine:	Outdoors

- Does your family spend much time outdoors? What do you do?
- What does your child do?
- Does your child like (the activity)?
- How does he get around?
- How does he interact with others?
- Are there any toys or games he engages with/in?
- How does your child let you know when he wants to do something different?
- What things does your child like or notice outside?
- Is this usually an enjoyable time? Would anything help make this time easier?
- What kinds of outdoor activities does he participate in? How much assistance does he need? How does he interact with his peers?

Notes	
Engagement	No information
Independence	No information
Social relationships	No information

Home: Satisfaction with routine (CIRCLE ONE)	*Classroom*: Fit of routine and child (CIRCLE ONE)
1. Not at all satisfied	1. Poor goodness of fit
2.	2.
3. Satisfied	3. Average goodness of fit
4.	4.
5. Very satisfied	5. Excellent goodness of fit

Domains addressed (CIRCLE ALL THAT APPLY):

Physical   Cognitive   Communication   Social or emotional   Adaptive

CHAPTER 3

Community-Based Everyday Child Learning Opportunities

CARL J. DUNST, MELINDA RAAB, CAROL M. TRIVETTE,
and JENNIFER SWANSON

The ways in which early childhood intervention for young children with disabilities and their families are conceptualized and implemented matters a great deal if both children and their parents are likely to realize optimal positive benefits. The three themes constituting the focus of this volume (everyday natural learning environments, normalized child and family experiences and opportunities, and capacity-building family involvement) taken together constitute contemporary thinking about how to produce such benefits. This includes but is not limited to child engagement, competence, and mastery, and parents' abilities to provide their children development-enhancing learning opportunities. This chapter includes the description of one way in which these themes can be operationalized and implemented. The focus of this chapter represents an approach to working with families of young children with disabilities that is intended to promote and support parent confidence and competence providing their children normalized learning opportunities as part of everyday community activities.

This chapter includes descriptions of the principles, practices, methods, and procedures for using everyday community activities as sources of development-enhancing child learning opportunities. Everyday community-based child learning activities include a rich array of formal and informal, structured and unstructured, and intentional and serendipitous learning opportunities, events, and experiences that provide infants, toddlers, and preschoolers contexts for practicing existing abilities and learning new capabilities (Dunst, Hamby, Trivette, Raab, & Bruder, 2000, 2002). Going to a twice-a-week parent–child play group is an example of a planned activity. Happening upon and getting to pet a puppy on a neighborhood walk is an example of an unplanned activity. Taking swimming lessons is an example of a structured activity. Kicking a soccer ball around the backyard is an example of an unstructured activity. Having a child brush his or her teeth after eating a meal or snack is an example of an intentional activity. Splashing in a puddle of water after a rainstorm is an example of a serendipitous learning activity.

The everyday community (as well as family) activities that are sources of child learning opportunities are natural environments (Dunst, Trivette, Humphries, Raab, & Roper, 2001). Natural learning environments are the settings where children learn context specific and both functional and adaptive skills that permit them to become increasingly more active participants in culturally relevant and meaningful activities (e.g., Alvarez, 1994; Chaiklin, Hedegaard, & Jensen, 1999; Ehrmann, Aeschleman, & Svanum, 1995; Tudge et al., 1999). Context specific, or situated learning (Chaiklin & Lave, 1996; Lave & Wenger, 1991), involves young children's acquisition and use of skills that "make sense" in the setting in which behavior is learned, practiced, and used to influence people and objects in those settings. The experiences afforded young children and their families as part of community life are viewed as those supports and resources that permit children with disabilities to become meaningfully involved in participatory learning opportunities (Jung, Chapter 1, this volume).

The particular approach to everyday community-based learning described in this chapter has evolved over a 25-year period of time from both research and practice (Dunst, 1981, 1985, 1992, 2001, 2006; Dunst & Shue, 2005; Trivette, Dunst, & Hamby, 2004). This research and practice has helped identify the sources of everyday child learning opportunities, patterns of child participation in those everyday activities, the characteristics and consequences of everyday development-enhancing child learning opportunities, the caregiver interactional styles that support child learning in everyday activities, and the child and caregiver benefits associated with participation in these kinds of learning activities. The "yield" from this research and practice has been the development of an approach to everyday child learning called Contextually Mediated Practices™ or CMP™ (Dunst, 2006; Dunst & Swanson, 2006). This chapter includes a description of this approach to early childhood intervention and tools (checklists and exhibits) for implementing CMP.

The chapter is divided into three sections. The first section includes a definition of early childhood intervention and four principles for implementing CMP. The second section includes an overview of the CMP model and the description of the key characteristics of this approach to early childhood intervention. The third section includes both a description of the methods and procedures for using CMP for supporting and strengthening both child and caregiver competence and confidence and checklists that practitioners can use for implementing CMP. The chapter concludes with a discussion of the factors that are likely to influence the adoption and use of CMP by early intervention, preschool special education, and other early childhood programs and practitioners working with young children with special needs and their families.

DEFINITION OF TERMS AND PRINCIPLES

The practices described in this chapter include an operational definition of early childhood intervention and four principles for defining the focus of CMP. Early childhood intervention is defined as

> *The everyday experiences and opportunities afforded infants, toddlers, and young children by the children's parents and other primary caregivers in the context of naturally occurring everyday learning activities that are intended to promote children's acquisition and use of behavioral competencies shaping and influencing prosocial interactions with people and materials.*

This definition emphasizes three key features of early childhood intervention: (1) the use of everyday activities as sources of child learning opportunities, (2) the parents' roles in facilitating and supporting child learning, and (3) the competency-enhancing outcomes that constitute measures of successful or effective early childhood intervention practices. The interested reader is referred to Dunst (2007) for a detailed description of the evidence supporting the use of these particular elements of early childhood intervention.

Guiding Principles

The approach to early childhood intervention constituting the focus of this chapter is based on four principles that guide the implementation of CMP. The principles, taken together, constitute a conceptual framework for operationalizing natural learning environment practices.

• *Principle 1. The everyday experiences used as sources of child learning opportunities should be ones that are culturally meaningful and which are contexts for mastering functional and socially adaptive behavioral competencies.* This principle is based on the contention that children's everyday lives are rich in learning opportunities (Dunst et al., 2000) and that these everyday activities are important contexts for child learning. The most important everyday activities are ones that are most meaningful in terms of increased child participation in family and community life and therefore by definition are context specific.

• *Principle 2. The experiences and opportunities afforded young children should strengthen children's self-initiated and self-directed learning and development promoting acquisition of functional behavioral competencies and children's recognition of their abilities to produce desired and expected effects and consequences.* A fundamental distinction is made between experiences and opportunities that are contexts for a child's acquisition and use of behavior that is intended to have desired child consequences (e.g., a child who learns to use a pointing gesture to have an adult retrieve a desired object) and those intended to elicit child behavior (e.g., having a child name objects shown to him or her by an adult). The former and not the latter is the type of early intervention practice constituting the focus of CMP.

• *Principle 3. Parent-mediated child learning is effective to the extent that it strengthens parents' confidence and competence in providing their children everyday development-instigating and development-enhancing learning opportunities and experiences.* This principle makes explicit that the benefits of early intervention should be realized by both children and their parents and other primary caregivers. The likelihood that parents and other primary caregivers will continue to provide their children the kinds of experiences and opportunities influencing development is maximized when adults recognize and understand the important role they play in influencing their children's growth and development (Goldberg, 1977).

• *Principle 4. The role of early childhood intervention practitioners in parent-mediated child learning is to support and strengthen parent capacity to provide their children experiences and opportunities of known qualities and characteristics (i.e., practices that are evidence-based) supporting and strengthening both child and parent competence and confidence.* Knowledgeable practitioners are aware of what research "tells us" about the characteristics of practices that are associated with optimal positive benefits (Dunst, Bruder, Trivette, & Hamby, 2006; Dunst, Trivette, Hamby, & Bruder, 2006). Practitioners intervene directly with children only to the extent that this serves a modeling role for parents to learn about and be able to use CMP with their children.

CAREGIVER-MEDIATED EVERYDAY CHILD LEARNING

Figure 3.1 shows the CMP model. The model includes four practice components (child interests, everyday activity settings, increased child learning opportunities, and parent-mediated child learning) and two major types of outcomes (activity setting participation and increased child and caregiver competence and confidence). The CMP model is used to promote parents' abilities to mediate children's participation in everyday activities increasing the number, frequency, and quality of interest-based child learning opportunities (Dunst & Swanson, 2006). Stated differently, the CMP model provides a foundation for parents and other primary caregivers to become more aware and capable of providing children a rich mix of learning opportunities as part of everyday life that are interesting, engaging, and motivating to their children, and which provide the children opportunities to practice existing abilities, learn new skills, and explore and learn about their own

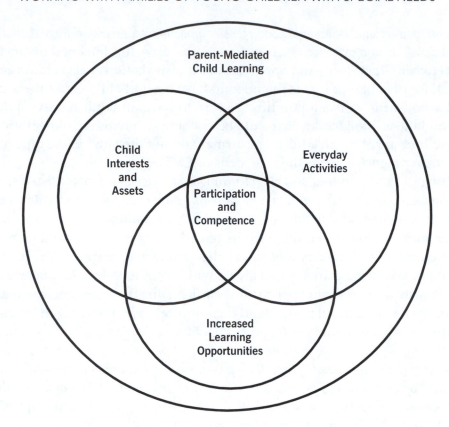

FIGURE 3.1. Major components of the Contextually Mediated Practices™ model for providing young children interest-based everyday learning opportunities.

capabilities as well as the propensities of others (e.g., the dependability of adults in the child's life). CMP is especially effective when implemented as part of working with families in the settings familiar and comfortable to them (R. A. McWilliam, Chapter 8, this volume).

Everyday Activity Settings

Children's lives throughout the world are made up of everyday activity settings that are contexts for child learning (see especially Göncü, 1999). Tharp and Gallimore (1988) defined everyday activity settings as the "contexts in which collaborative interaction, intersubjectivity, assisted performance, and learning occurs" (p. 72). Farver (1999) noted that "activity settings are made up of everyday experiences . . . [that] . . . contain ordinary settings in which children's social interaction and behavior occurs. They are the who, what, where, when, and why of daily life" (p. 201).

Activity settings that are part of everyday *community* life include, but are not limited to, car, subway, or bus rides; eating out; neighborhood walks; hiking; library story time hours; play groups; feeding ducks or fish at a community pond; restaurant playlands; and so forth (Beckman et al., 1998; Dunst, 2000; Dunst & Hamby, 1999a; Dunst, Hamby, Trivette, Raab, & Bruder, 2000; Gallimore, Goldenberg, & Weisner, 1993; Hatcher & Beck, 1997). Activity settings that are part of everyday *family life* include such things as dressing and undressing, eating meals, brushing teeth, taking care of pets, getting ready for bed, roughhousing, parent–child play episodes, household chores, and so forth (Dunst & Hamby, 1999b; Dunst et al., 2000; Gallimore, Weisner, Bernheimer, Guthrie, & Nihira, 1993; Gallimore, Weisner, Kaufman, & Bernheimer, 1989; Lamb, Leyendecker, Schölmerich, & Fracasso, 1998; Tudge et al., 1999). In a national study of parents of infants, toddlers, and preschoolers, Dunst et al. (2000) identified 11 categories of community activities and 11 categories of family activities that were sources of everyday child learning. Table 3.1 shows the categories of everyday community activities identified in this study and the kinds of learning opportunities that can happen in the activities. This table can be especially helpful in understanding the scope of everyday community learning activities and can be used as part of completing a checklist for identifying everyday activities that are sources for interest-based child learning opportunities (see below).

Learning opportunities afforded young children as part of everyday community (and family) life can be either contextualized or decontextualized (Lave, 1996). The difference between contextualized and decontextualized learning opportunities is illustrated by the following examples. A child walking up or down steps in order to go outside to play is an example of a contextual learning opportunity, whereas a child repeatedly going up or down steps to "practice weight shifting" is an example of a noncontextual learning opportunity. A child using gestures, signs, or words to request something to eat at mealtimes is an example of a contextual learning opportunity, whereas a child repeating the words for foods shown in pictures or on flash cards is an example of a noncontextual learning opportunity. A child getting an adult to play "pat-a-cake" by pushing the adult's hands together is an example of a contextual learning opportunity, whereas having a child repeatedly imitate gestures or repeatedly make hand or arm movements is an example of a noncontextual learning opportunity. A child making swimming strokes or "doggy paddling" as part of taking swimming lessons is an example of a contextualized learning opportunity, whereas doing range-of-motion exercises while in a swimming pool is an example of a noncontextualized learning opportunity.

The distinction between contextualized and decontextualized learning helps clarify when experiences afforded young children are and are not the kinds of everyday natural learning opportunities that are most valued and desired. Simply stated, "learning opportunities provided in the context of everyday activities are the most desired natural learning opportunities when the learning itself is functional and socially adaptive." Consequently, "moving" decontextualized learning opportunities out of clinics or other nonnormative places into community and family activity settings does not make the change in location natural learning opportunities.

TABLE 3.1. Categorization of Everyday Community Learning Opportunities

Category/examples	*Category*/examples	*Category*/examples
Family activities	*Clubs/organizations*	*Outdoor activities*
Getting groceries	Attending dance classes	Beach activities
Helping at laundromat	Attending ethnic/heritage clubs	Bird watching
Helping with community	Attending gymnastics/movement	Boating/canoeing
clean-up	classes	Camping
Paying bills with parent	Attending music classes	Hiking
Picking up siblings from school	Baby exercise classes	Kite flying
Recycling	Going to 4H clubs	Nature trail walks
Running errands	Going to arts and crafts classes	Planting a community garden
Taking car/bus/train rides	Going to hobby/activity clubs	Rafting
	Mommy and Me playgroups	
Family outings	Playful Parenting	*Amusements/attractions*
Collecting leaves/rocks	Scouting/Campfire Girls/Indian	Attending a circus
Eating out	Guides	Going to an aquarium
Going on neighborhood walks	Taking martial arts classes	Going to a nature preserve
Going to family reunions		Going to a pumpkin patch
Going to holiday gatherings	*Parks/recreation activities*	Petting animals at petting zoos
Having picnics/cookouts	Attending open/family gym time	Visiting amusement or theme
Shopping at mall/supermarket	Biking	parks
Visiting friends/neighbors	Bowling	Visiting animal farms
Visiting parent at work	Family tennis	Visiting aviaries
	Fishing	Visiting historic sites
Play activities	Horseback riding	Visiting pet stores/animal
Attending baby/toddler gym	Skating	shelters
Attending child care/preschools	Skiing	Watching animals at a zoo or
groups	Sledding	wildlife preserve
Attending child play groups	Snowmobiling	
Dodgeball	Swimming	*Sports activities*
Kickball	Track/running	Cheerleading
Neighborhood hiding games		Playing baseball/t-ball
Playing at indoor playlands	*Community events*	Playing basketball
Playing on playground	Attending ceremonial events	Playing golf/miniature golf
sandboxes/slides/climbers	Attending community Easter Egg	Playing soccer
Playing with animals/pets	hunts	Watching car races
	Attending community	Watching football games
Art/entertainment activities	gatherings/rallies	Watching hockey
Attending library/bookstore	Attending community hayrides	
story hours	Attending family festivals/events	*Religious activities*
Attending music concerts	Attending farm shows	Attending baptisms
Attending puppet shows	Attending fireworks displays/	Attending church fundraisers
Going to an art show	light shows	Attending church socials/
Going to Ice Capades	Going to street fairs	gatherings
Listening to storytellers	Local/county/regional fairs (face	Attending church/synagogue
Seeing a magic show	painting, children's rides)	Attending religious ceremonies
Seeing movies	Watching historical	Attending Sunday school
Visiting a children's museum	reenactments/celebrations	Attending Vacation Bible school
Visiting planetariums	Watching parades	Attending weddings
Visiting a science center		Going to religion classes
Watching a children's play/		Playing at church nursery
musical		
Watching a dance performance		

One very important point needs to be made about the everyday activities infants, toddlers, and preschoolers experience as part of community (as well as family) life. Many of the activities that young children experience are often ones where their involvement is indirect or peripheral but where they nonetheless benefit behaviorally and developmentally (see especially Lave & Wenger, 1991). Everyday activities that young children are involved in often include adult activities (e.g., Rogoff, Mosier, Mistry, & Göncü, 1993) or the activities of older children (e.g., Lancy, 1996) that draw infants, toddlers, and preschoolers into interactions with people and materials that provide contexts for many different kinds of learning opportunities. Tagging along to an older sibling's T-ball game where a toddler is afforded opportunities to play with baseballs, "run" the bases, attempt to swing a bat, and clap and cheer at his sister making a hit are examples of these peripheral learning opportunities. Many of the everyday activities included in Table 3.1 are these kinds of learning opportunities. Practitioners using the checklist with a parent therefore should be aware of the potential learning opportunities afforded by "tag-along" activities and other activities in which a child is a secondary participant.

Child Interests

Learning in general, and child learning more specifically, are likely to be maximized if the learning is interest-based, engaging, and motivating to the learner (Raab & Dunst, 2007; Renninger, 1998). Interests include the likes, preferences, favorites, strengths, assets, and so forth that motivate children (as well as adults) to engage and participate in desired activities providing contexts for both interest and competence expression. Interests are either or both a *person* or *environment* (*situational*) characteristic (Krapp, Hidi, & Renninger, 1992; Raab, 2005). Personal interests include a child's personal likes, preferences, favorites, strengths, and so forth. Situational interests include those aspects of social and nonsocial environments that attract child attention, curiosity, and engagement in interactions with people and objects. According to Renninger, Hidi, and Krapp (1992), both personal and situational interests influence child learning and development. Research shows that both types of interest-based child learning opportunities are associated with increased positive and decreased negative child behavior and functioning (Raab & Dunst, 2007). Interest-based child participation in everyday activities functions as a type of positive behavior support emphasizing child production of prosocial behavior (Fox, Chapter 9, this volume).

The framework shown in Figure 3.2 guides the implementation of CMP and includes the key features of everyday learning opportunities that mirror what we know from available research. The foundation of the model is interest-based child learning opportunities that occur in the context of everyday activities. Research indicates that children's learning is enhanced when interests engage children in social and nonsocial interactions with people and objects that provide opportuni-

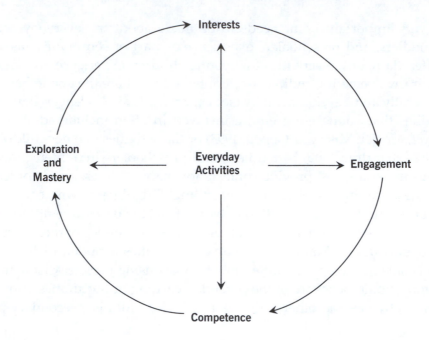

FIGURE 3.2. Everyday activity settings as sources of interest-based and competence-enhancing everyday natural learning opportunities.

ties to practice existing skills, explore their social and nonsocial environments, and learn and master new abilities (Raab & Dunst, 2007). Nelson (1999), for example, found that variations in the development of children's language competence were "related easily to the child's life activities and interests" (p. 2). Similarly, Guberman (1999) noted, "children's own interests and sense-making processes [are] a central formulation of supportive [learning] environments" (p. 207).

The way in which interests function as either a person or environment factor (Bronfenbrenner, 1993; Wachs, 2000) influencing child learning and development can be explained as follows. People, objects, and events that are either a child's personal interests or things that are interesting to a child are likely to capture and maintain the child's attention (Fogel, 1997), encourage the child to interact with people and objects (Rusher, Cross, & Ware, 1995), and promote child participation in social and nonsocial activities (Göncü, Tuermer, Jain, & Johnson, 1999). Interest-based playing and interaction provide the foundation for increased child engagement (McWilliam & Ware, 1994). When a child is engaged in everyday activities, the activities provide opportunities to practice existing abilities, perfect emerging skills, and acquire new competence (Farver, 1999). Everyday activities that afford a child opportunities to display competence are ones that are more likely to encourage and support exploration (Wachs, 1979). Through exploration, a child learns the relationship between his or her behavior and its consequences, both enhancing and strengthening a sense of mastery (MacTurk & Morgan, 1995). A sense of mastery in turn is likely to reinforce existing interests and promote the development of new ones.

Increasing Child Learning Opportunities

Participation in everyday activities can only have positive effects on learning and development if children have a sufficient *number of opportunities* to participate in different kinds of social and nonsocial activities having development-instigating and development-enhancing qualities (Bronfenbrenner, 1992, 1993). According to Bronfenbrenner (1999), "For development to occur, the [developing] person must engage in activity . . . and the activity must take place on a fairly regular basis" (pp. 5–6). The importance of opportunity derives from the simple fact that engagement in everyday activity provides a child opportunities to practice existing capabilities as well as learn new capabilities (Bourdieu, 1977; Lave, 1996). According to Duchan (1997), the "goal of a situated [contextual] approach to [therapy and intervention] focuses on increasing opportunities for . . . a child to participate in everyday-life activities" (p. 10). Consequently, *increasing the number, frequency, and quality of opportunities for children to participate in interest-based everyday activity* is a primary focus of CMP.

Child learning opportunities are increased by both participation in different kinds of interest-based everyday activities and by the number of learning opportunities afforded in any one everyday activity. Take, for example, a child who enjoys playing in water. Getting to play in water during bath time, using a hose to water plants and flowers, splashing in a puddle of water, and dropping pebbles in a stream or pond, are examples of interest-based participation in different kinds of everyday activity. Splashing in a wading pool, floating things in the pool, filling and emptying a bucket of pool water, and pretending to swim in the pool are examples of different kinds of interest-based learning opportunities in the same everyday activity. Increasing both the *breadth* and *depth* of interest-based everyday activities is a major focus of CMP.

Parent-Mediated Child Learning

Parent-mediated child learning involves the *intentional* use of different methods and strategies for recognizing, identifying, and acknowledging child interests and abilities; using this information for engaging children in interest-based everyday learning activities; and encouraging and supporting children's learning and competence expression in the context of the everyday activities. This is accomplished using a number of different practices where CMP *is most likely to benefit both a child and parent when a parent is the primary or principal agent providing a child interest-based everyday learning opportunities*. Research indicates, for example, that parenting competence is strengthened when parents use everyday activities as sources of child learning opportunities and children demonstrate positive functioning in the activities (Dunst, Bruder et al., 2006).

Mediation includes three different components or processes: planning, implementation, and evaluation and feedback. *Planning* involves child interest identification and decisions about which everyday activities are the best contexts for interest-based child learning. *Implementation* involves parents' efforts to increase child participation in different everyday activities and what parents do to support and encourage child learning in those activities. *Evaluation and feedback* involve parent appraisals of whether his or her child benefited from the everyday learning opportunities and the extent to which his or her efforts to support child learning were successful. The section of the chapter below describing how to use CMP for providing children interest-based everyday learning opportunities includes methods and procedures for planning, implementing, and evaluating the CMP caregiver-mediated approach to early childhood intervention.

Outcomes and Benefits

CMP is judged successful to the extent that children have increased opportunities to participate in socially and culturally meaningful everyday activities, and both child and parent competence and confidence are strengthened as a consequence of parent-mediated child learning. *Participation* refers to the ways in which a child takes part in an everyday activity—beginning it, ending it, joining in interactions, giving and asking for assistance, and so forth—promoting involvement in the social and cultural activities, experiences, and opportunities that are valued by the family (Shweder et al., 1998). Child participation is considered successful to the extent that everyday activities provide opportunities to learn, practice, and perfect abilities permitting a child to "fit" into his or her social and cultural groups and settings.

Several different aspects of *child and parent competence* constitute the desired outcomes of CMP. *Child competence* includes the behavior children use to initiate and sustain interactions with and feedback from people and objects. These child-initiated and self-directed behaviors are described as interactive competencies (Dunst, Holbert, & Wilson, 1990; Dunst & McWilliam, 1988). An interactive competency is a child behavior that is used to produce environmental consequences demonstrating a *shift in balance of power* in interactions with people (and objects) toward the developing child. A shift in balance of power is manifested in situations when a child initiates more interactions than do their parents or other primary caregivers in an everyday activity, and they attempt to prosocially and proactively "control" the nature or content of interactions with people and objects in those activities (e.g., Bronfenbrenner, 1979). Dunst (1979), for example, found that children either with or without disabilities showed this type of shift in balance of power between 8 and 14 months of age developmentally in interactions with their mothers.

Parent competence includes parents' abilities to identify child interests, select everyday activities as contexts of interest expression, increase child participation in everyday activities, and support child learning in these activities. Special attention is placed on caregiver self-efficacy beliefs that are known to be mediators of other kinds of parenting behavior (see especially Dunst, Trivette, & Hamby, 2006, 2008). These self-efficacy beliefs are assessed in terms of parents' judgments about their abilities to plan and provide their children interest-based everyday learning opportunities that lead to desired outcomes (Bandura, 1997).

Child and parent confidence also constitute the focus of evaluating CMP. Confidence is assessed in terms of behavioral indicators that are measures of a sense of accomplishment and positive feelings about one's own behavioral capabilities. Child confidence includes smiling, laughter, verbalizations, excitement, and so forth manifested in response to producing desired behavioral effects or consequences (Dunst, Raab et al., 2007; Trevarthen & Hubley, 1978). Caregiver confidence includes the gratification derived from providing child development-enhancing learning opportunities and the recognition of child benefits from these experiences (Goldberg, 1977; Okagaki & Divecha, 1993).

IMPLEMENTING AND PRACTICING CMP

CMP is implemented by parents and other primary caregivers using methods and procedures for (1) identifying children's interests and the everyday community and family activities that constitute the makeup of a child's life, (2) selecting those activities that provide the best opportunities for interest-based learning, (3) increasing child participation in interest-based everyday learning opportunities, (4) using different interactional techniques for supporting and encouraging child competence, exploration, and mastery in the activities, and (5) evaluating the effectiveness of parent-mediated everyday child learning opportunities in terms of both child and parent benefits (Dunst, 2006; Dunst & Swanson, 2006). The results from efforts to promote child participation and learning using CMP are also used to make decisions about those interest-based everyday activities that are continued, discontinued, or modified. CMP is one of a number of approaches to early childhood intervention that are implemented in the contexts of everyday activities and routines (R. A. McWilliam, Chapter 2, this volume).

Figure 3.3 shows the manner in which CMP is implemented by parents and other primary caregivers. The *planning phase* of CMP involves either the selection of everyday activities that are likely to be interesting to a child or the use of information about child interests to select everyday activities that can be used as contexts for interest expression. The *implementation phase* involves parents' intentional efforts to increase the number, frequency, and quality of interest-based everyday child learning opportunities, parent responsiveness to child behavior in interest-

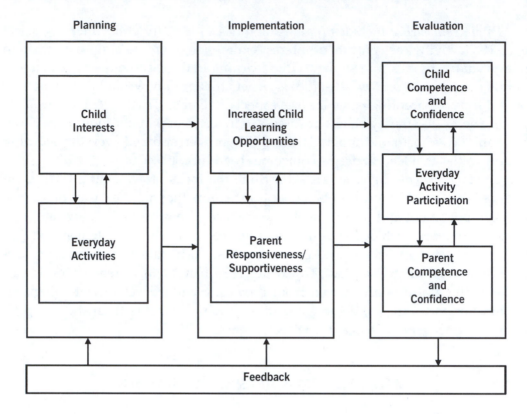

FIGURE 3.3. Process for planning, implementing, and evaluating the effectiveness of CMP.

based everyday activities, and parents' efforts to support and encourage child competence, exploration, and mastery. The *evaluation phase* of CMP involves measures of both child and parent benefits of everyday child learning. The *feedback phase* involves the use of evaluative information by a parent for changing existing or developing new everyday learning opportunities. All phases of implementation are accomplished using effective communication skills (P. J. McWilliam, Chapter 5, this volume) that are culturally sensitive and respectful of parental beliefs and values (Hanson & Lynch, Chapter 6, this volume).

Five checklists are used to facilitate practitioners' abilities to promote caregivers' use of parent-mediated child learning. Table 3.2 shows the recommended sequence in which the checklists are used for implementing CMP. The checklists are used to identify child interests, select everyday activities that are contexts for interest-based child learning, increase child participation in those activities, support and encourage child competence as part of interest-based learning opportunities, and determine the effectiveness of parent-mediated child learning opportunities. The particular focus of the checklists is participation in everyday community activities although the broader-based CMP model includes participation in both family and community activities (Dunst, 2006; Dunst & Swanson, 2006). The check-

TABLE 3.2. Checklists for Promoting Caregiver Use of Parent-Mediated Child Learning

Sequence	Checklists	Main focus
1	Child Interests	Child personal and situational interests, preferences, etc.
2	Everyday Community Learning Activities	Types and sources of everyday community learning activities
3	Increasing Everyday Child Learning Opportunities	Increasing the number, frequency, and quality of interest-based learning activities
4	Caregiver Responsive Teaching	Methods for supporting and encouraging child learning in everyday activities
5	Parent-Mediated Child Learning Evaluation	Measuring the success of CMP

lists were developed specifically to support what a practitioner can do to promote parents' and other primary caregivers' adoption and use of CMP. The checklists are included in Appendices 3.1–3.5 at the end of this chapter.

Planning

Parents and other primary caregivers are especially good at knowing and recognizing their children's likes and dislikes, preferred and nonpreferred activities, and their strengths and weaknesses. The intentional use of this information for identifying the particular everyday activities that provide the best contexts for interest-based learning is fundamentally important as part of providing children interest-based everyday natural learning opportunities.

Child Interests

Identifying child interests is accomplished using the Child Interests Checklist (Appendix 3.1). The procedures for assessing the presence of child interests are straightforward and include answers to questions such as What does the child like? What makes the child smile and laugh? What captures and maintains the child's attention? What kinds of things does the child prefer or like to do? and so forth. The answers to these questions will produce a profile of a child's interests, assets, strengths, preferences, and so forth that in turn are used to select everyday activities that are the best contexts for interest-based learning. Interest-based child learning simply includes opportunities to do what a child likes, prefers to do, and enjoys doing. Table 3.3 includes a list of sources readers may find helpful for identifying both personal and situational child interests.

TABLE 3.3. Methods for Identifying Child Interests

Dunst, C. J., Herter, S., & Shields, H. (2000). Interest-based natural learning opportunities. In S. Sandall & M. Ostrosky (Eds.), *Natural environments and inclusion* (Young Exceptional Children Monograph Series No. 2, pp. 37–48). Longmont, CO: Sopris West.

Dunst, C. J., Roberts, K., & Snyder, D. (2004). *Spotting my child's very special interests: A workbook for parents.* Asheville, NC: Winterberry Press.

Dunst, C. J., & Snyder, D. (2004). *Possibilities interest assessment interview protocol.* Asheville, NC: Winterberry Press.

Orelena Hawks Puckett Institute (Producer). (2004). *Spotting my child's very special interests: A guide for parents* [Visual recording]. Asheville, NC: Winterberry Press.

Raab, M. (2005). Interest-based child participation in everyday learning activities. *CASEinPoint, 1*(2), 1–5. Available at *www.fippcase.org/caseinpoint/caseinpoint_vol1_ no2.pdf.*

Community Activities

The everyday community (as well as family) activities that are candidates for interest-based child learning will vary by child age, where a child lives, parents' beliefs and values, and so forth. Table 3.1 above provides examples of the kinds of everyday community activities that many children experience as part of everyday community life. The Everyday Community Learning Activity Checklist (Appendix 3.2) was developed specifically to provide practitioners a way to help parents and other primary caregivers select from all possible kinds of community activities those that will provide a child *variety* (breadth) and *richness* (depth) in the learning activities that best match a child's interests and therefore are likely to be contexts for strengthening existing capabilities and promoting acquisition of new competencies. Table 3.4 includes other sources that readers may want to examine for additional ideas about everyday community activities.

TABLE 3.4. Methods for Identifying Everyday Community Learning Activities

Dunst, C. J., & Hamby, D. (1999). Community life as sources of children's learning opportunities. *Children's Learning Opportunities Report, 1*(4). Available at *www. everydaylearning.info/reports/lov1-4.pdf*

Dunst, C. J., Herter, S., Shields, H., & Bennis, L. (2001). Mapping community-based natural learning opportunities. *Young Exceptional Children, 4*(4), 16–24.

Dunst, C. J., & Shue, P. (2005). Creating literacy-rich natural learning environments for infants, toddlers, and preschoolers. In E. M. Horn & H. Jones (Eds.), *Supporting early literacy development in young children* (Young Exceptional Children Monograph Series No. 7, pp. 15–30). Longmont, CO: Sopris West.

Orelena Hawks Puckett Institute (Producer). (2001). *Power of the ordinary: A photographic journey of children's everyday learning opportunities* [Visual recording]. Asheville, NC: Winterberry Press.

Orelena Hawks Puckett Institute (Producer). (2002). *Anyplace, anytime, anywhere! Everyday learning in community activities* (Natural Learning Opportunities Video Series No. 2) [Video tape]. Asheville, NC: Winterberry Press.

Selecting Interest-Based Learning Opportunities

The main outcome of the planning phase of CMP is the selection of between 8 and 10 everyday activities that parents or other caregivers consider the learning opportunities that will occur frequently enough to provide a child a host of different kinds of interest-based learning opportunities. The process for doing so is straightforward. A practitioner helps a parent select from all possible activities those that match child interests, happen frequently enough to ensure sufficient numbers of learning opportunities, and provide lots of opportunities as part of any one activity to practice existing capabilities, learn new behaviors, and otherwise encourage child exploration. The activities that are selected from all possibilities are then used as part of the implementation phase of CMP.

Implementation

Implementation of CMP involves increased child participation in interest-based everyday learning opportunities and caregivers' use of responsive teaching techniques for supporting and encouraging child competence in the activities. The following example illustrates what this looks like and how it is accomplished. A child with a particular interest in animals is taken to a community pond by his father three or four times a week. The child especially likes feeding the ducks at the pond. The son and father take a bag of breadcrumbs to the pond and the father hands the crumbs to his son who "throws" them at a paddle of ducks. The excitement the ducks show is especially engaging to the young child. He "asks" for more breadcrumbs by holding out his hand to his father to continue the feeding episode. The father at every opportunity responds to the child's behavior by showing excitement, by talking about what his son is doing, and by encouraging his son to actively engage in asking for more breadcrumbs, feeding and reaching for the ducks, repeating quacking sounds, and using simple words to describe what he sees he is doing.

Efforts to have parents increase their children's participation in everyday activities and use interactional styles that are known to strengthen and promote child competence have proven quite easy. In one study, for example, it took less than 2 weeks for parents to increase the number, frequency, and variety of everyday child learning opportunities (Dunst, Bruder et al., 2001). It was similarly easy to encourage parents' use of simple, but highly effective interactional styles for supporting child learning in the activities.

Increasing Child Learning Opportunities

In order for CMP to be optimally effective, the number, frequency, and variety of everyday community activities need to be sufficiently increased to provide a child breadth and depth in learning opportunities. The Increasing Everyday Child Learn-

TABLE 3.5. Methods for Increasing Child Participation in Everyday Learning Activities

Dunst, C. J. (2001). Participation of young children with disabilities in community learning activities. In M. J. Guralnick (Ed.), *Early childhood inclusion: Focus on change* (pp. 307–333). Baltimore: Brookes.

Dunst, C. J. (2008). *Parent and community assets as sources of young children's learning opportunities* (Revised and expanded ed.). Asheville, NC: Winterberry Press.

Raab, M., & Dunst, C. J. (2006). Checklists for promoting parent-mediated everyday child learning opportunities. *CASEtools, 2*(1), 1–9. Available at *www.fippcase.org/casetools/casetools_vol2_no1.pdf*.

Swanson, J., Raab, M., Roper, N., & Dunst, C. J. (2006). Promoting young children's participation in interest-based everyday learning activities. *CASEtools, 2*(5), 1–22. Available at *www.fippcase.org/casetools/casetools_vol2_no5.pdf*.

---

ing Opportunities Checklist (Appendix 3.3) includes practices that can be used for increasing participation in everyday community learning activities. Increasing child participation in interest-based everyday community learning activities is accomplished using any number of "reminders" that parents can use to facilitate the provision of everyday learning opportunities. These include, but are not limited to, a daily reminder list of activities (something like a shopping list), a weekly calendar, or an activity schedule (see, e.g., Dunst, Lesko, et al., 1987) that prompts a parent to engage the child in the activities selected in the planning phase of CMP. The goal is to increase the *breadth* and *depth* of participation in everyday community learning opportunities. The reader should also find the sources included in Table 3.5 useful in terms of other ways this can be accomplished.

Caregiver Responsiveness

What parents do to support and encourage child learning as part of children's participation in everyday activities is important for a number of reasons. Research indicates that parent responsiveness to and support of child behavior in the context of everyday activities is a potent strategy for supporting and strengthening child competence expression and for promoting child acquisition of new abilities (Dunst & Kassow, 2008; Kassow & Dunst, 2007a, b; Nievar & Becker, 2008; Shonkoff & Phillips, 2000). Responsive teaching, incidental teaching, and other *in vivo* instructional techniques and strategies emphasizing responsiveness to and support of child competence expression are especially effective when children are engaged in interaction with people and objects (see e.g., Dunst, Lowe, & Bartholomew, 1990).

The Caregiver Responsive Teaching Checklist (Appendix 3.4) includes those aspects of this approach to teaching that support interest-based learning and child competence and confidence. The checklist includes practices for focusing caregiver attention on child interests, responding contingently to child behavior, encouraging child production of new behavior, and providing the child opportunities to practice and perfect newly learned behavior. The practices taken together constitute an interactional style that has been found especially effective as a teaching method for supporting and strengthening child competence and confidence as part of partici-

TABLE 3.6. Descriptions of Caregiver Responsive Teaching

Orelena Hawks Puckett Institute (Producer). (2005). *Tune in: Responsive interaction style* [Visual recording]. Asheville, NC: Winterberry Press.

Roberts, K. (2007). *Pathways to parent–child closeness: Research findings show the best kinds of interactions* (Winterberry Research Summaries Vol. 1, No. 23). Asheville, NC: Winterberry Press.

Roberts, K. (2007). *Research reveals practical pointers for beneficial adult–child interaction* (Winterberry Research Summaries Vol. 1, No. 12). Asheville, NC: Winterberry Press.

Roberts, K. (2007). *Sense and sensitivity: Research indicates best ways to boost parental sensitivity to child behavior* (Winterberry Research Summaries Vol. 1, No. 13). Asheville, NC: Winterberry Press.

pation in interest-based everyday learning activities (Dunst & Kassow, 2008; Kassow & Dunst, 2007a; Trivette, 2007). Many of the key features of parental support, responsiveness, and encouragement of child learning in everyday community (as well as family) activities can be found in the sources included in Table 3.6.

Evaluation

CMP is successful to the extent that a child has increased opportunities to participate in interest-based everyday community (as well as family) activities, child competence and confidence is strengthened as a result of participation in everyday learning activities, and parents' competence and confidence is strengthened as a result of their efforts to provide their children interest-based everyday learning opportunities. The Parent-Mediated Child Learning Evaluation Checklist (Appendix 3.5) includes the outcomes that are considered most important in measuring the effectiveness of this approach to early childhood intervention. Table 3.7 includes sources of information on evaluation tools that practitioners should find helpful as well.

Child Everyday Activity Participation

Increased participation in everyday activities is determined by asking parents whether a child's participation in the activities identified in the planning phase

TABLE 3.7. Procedures for Evaluating the Effectiveness of CMP

Dunst, C. J., & Masiello, T. L. (2003). *Everyday parenting scale (modified version)*. Asheville, NC: Winterberry Press.

Dunst, C. J., Raab, M., Trivette, C. M., Parkey, C., Gatens, M., Wilson, L. L., et al. (2007). Child and adult social–emotional benefits of response-contingent child learning opportunities. *Journal of Early and Intensive Behavior Intervention, 4*, 379-391.

Dunst, C. J., & Trivette, C. M. (2003). *Child learning opportunities scale*. Asheville, NC: Winterberry Press.

Trivette, C. M., & Dunst, C. J. (2004). Evaluating family-based practices: Parenting experiences scale. *Young Exceptional Children, 7*(3), 12–19.

has increased, remained the same, or has decreased since using CMP. The extent to which participation in the activities is interest-based and the activities have development-enhancing qualities is determined by asking parents to assess the characteristics of the learning opportunities (e.g., Dunst & Trivette, 2003). This is determined, for example, by asking parents to indicate the extent to which the learning activities were interest-based (e.g., "child got excited while engaged in the activities"), maintained the child's attention (e.g., "the activities maintained the child's attention"), provided opportunities for competence expression (e.g., "child tried his/her hardest during the activities"), and strengthened a child's ability to initiate and sustain the games (e.g., "child tried to start or initiate interactions in the activities") (Dunst, Pace, & Hamby, 2007; Trivette, Dunst, Hamby, & Pace, 2007).

Child Benefits

Child competence is assessed by observations of child behavior that would be expected to be the consequence of interest-based child learning opportunities. This is accomplished for each everyday activity by recording those behaviors that the child uses in interactions with the people, objects, and materials in those settings. Child confidence is assessed in terms of a sense of self-efficacy and accomplishment in achieving desired effects or producing expected consequences. The behavior indicators of confidence include, but are not limited to, social-affective behavior (smiling, laughter, vocalizations) and excitement demonstrated as part of or in response to producing desired or expected consequences (Dunst, Raab et al., 2007).

Caregiver Benefits

Parenting confidence and competence are measured using any number of behavioral indicators in which the instructions are written in terms of the extent to which CMP has had an effect on parenting behavior or beliefs (e.g., "To what extent has your use of CMP made you feel more capable about the learning opportunities you have been providing your child?"). Competence is assessed in terms of caregiver capabilities to execute parenting roles (e.g., providing a child interest-based learning opportunities), and confidence is assessed in terms of the sense of accomplishment in having expected or anticipated consequences (e.g., increasing child production of context-specific functional behavior).

Feedback

The extent to which parents and other primary caregivers continue to provide their children everyday learning opportunities and support their children's production of competence in the activities is dependent on the self-efficacy evaluations of their parent-mediated efforts. Two types of self-efficacy belief appraisals (Bandura, 1997) are likely to influence parents' attributions and actions: (1) the extent to which the learning opportunities afforded a child have expected or desired child consequences, and (2) the extent to which the parents' decisions and actions strengthen their own confidence and competence in their parenting capabilities.

The information obtained in the evaluation phase of CMP is used to engage parents in discussion, reflection, and self-evaluation of their actions as a way of deciding to continue, discontinue, modify, change, and so forth the activities afforded their children. The importance of doing so is based on research showing that parents' self-efficacy beliefs are important mediators of both the experiences afforded children and the benefits and consequences of the experiences for their children (e.g., Coleman & Karraker, 2003; Coleman et al., 2002; Dunst, Trivette, & Hamby, 2006; Teti & Gelfand, 1991). Parents and other primary caregivers are more likely to continue providing their children interest-based everyday learning opportunities if they judge their efforts successful in increasing child participation in the activities and the observed or experienced benefits of their participation include both child and parent competence and confidence.

CONCLUSION

The extent to which practitioners are likely to use CMP to promote parents' understanding and use of parent-mediated everyday child learning opportunities is dependent on a number of factors and conditions. First, practitioners need to recognize the importance of both everyday community (as well as family) activities as sources of child learning opportunities and the roles parents and other primary caregivers play in supporting child learning in those activities. Second, practitioners need to value and derive gratification from seeing parents become increasingly more capable of providing their children development-enhancing learning opportunities. Third, practitioners need to recognize and adopt asset- and strengths-based models for supporting both parent and child confidence and competence in order to maximize the benefits of CMP. Finally, practitioners need to recognize that practitioner-implemented interventions once or even twice a week in the absence of parent-mediated child learning accounts for so small an amount of learning opportunities that the likelihood of making a meaningful difference in terms of child outcomes and benefits is minimal at best (Dunst, 2006, 2007; McWilliam, 2000).

The likelihood of parents and other caregivers adopting and using CMP for promoting child learning is dependent on a number of factors and conditions as well. First, parents need to recognize the important role they play in providing their children everyday interest-based learning opportunities. Second, parents need to value child-initiated learning and recognize the fact that increases in child-initiated behavior are important indicators of child competence. Third, parents need to understand that the manner in which they support and encourage child learning matters a great deal in terms of both child and parent benefits. Finally, parents need to expect and demand that practitioners not take over caregiving functions so that they do not have negative effects on parents' sense of their own capabilities (Dunst, Bruder et al., 2006; Dunst, Trivette, Hamby et al., 2006; Hewlett & West, 1998).

The approach to early childhood intervention described in this chapter is one of a number of ways of implementing natural learning environment practices (see, e.g., R. A. McWilliam, Chapter 2, this volume). We consider CMP the approach of choice for providing young children interest-based everyday community (as well as family) learning opportunities, because there are positive effects associated with interest-based child learning opportunities and negative effects associated with practitioners implementing interventions in everyday community (as well as family) activities (Dunst, Brookfield, & Epstein, 1998; Dunst, Bruder et al., 2001; Dunst, Bruder et al., 2006; Dunst, Hamby, & Brookfield, 2007; Dunst, Trivette, & Cutspec, 2007; Dunst, Trivette, Hamby et al., 2006; Janes & Kermani, 2001). This observation, as well as other research, provides the empirical foundation for a parent-mediated approach to early childhood intervention despite the fact that the use of this approach to natural learning environment practices has, for the most part, not been adopted by many practitioners (Dunst & Raab, 2004; Raab & Dunst, 2004).

Several factors appear to account for the reason why CMP-type intervention practices are not used widely by early childhood intervention practitioners, and especially practitioners working in Individuals with Disabilities Education Act (IDEA) Part C early intervention programs. One factor is the lack of practitioner understanding of the meaning of natural learning environments and the conditions under which everyday learning opportunities are likely to have optimal positive child and parent benefits. CMP is deceptively simple and its commonsense features seem to be a factor that interferes with its adoption. Practitioners as well as parents often overlook the value and importance of everyday learning since it is not formalized and often does not appear to be intervention despite evidence to the contrary.

A second factor is the increased use of Medicaid funding by IDEA Part C early intervention programs and providers, especially in states where practitioners are not reimbursed for their services unless they directly work with children. This more often than not results in the provision of decontextualized, nonfunctional services, which, as noted above, is more likely to be disruptive to parents and children.

A third factor is the disconnect between research and practice, and especially research findings that run counter to commonly held beliefs about what constitutes "best practices." To say that early childhood intervention practice has not kept pace with research is an understatement (see, especially, Dunst, 2007). Early childhood intervention with young children with disabilities or delays, as currently practiced for the most part, is characterized by elements and features that research tells us cannot make much of a difference in a child's life.

The possibility of practices described in this chapter being widely used by programs and practitioners requires considerable rethinking about the methods and goals of early childhood intervention. This is likely to occur only when practitioners become increasingly aware of practices that work and do not work, and practitioners engage in thoughtful reflection about how to change or improve them. The content of the chapter lays the groundwork for this rethinking and includes concrete things practitioners can do to become evidence-based practitioners. The methods and procedures for implementing CMP should therefore prove informative and useful to practitioners who strive to provide young children the kinds of learning opportunities that are likely to matter most in terms of both child and caregiver benefits.

We conclude by noting the fact that parents' abilities to use CMP or any other kind of practice is dependent on whether they have the time and energy to carry out parenting roles and responsibilities. CMP is a component of family systems intervention (Dunst, 2004; Dunst & Trivette, 2008), where parents and other family member concerns and priorities are addressed so that they have the physical and psychological energy to engage their children in everyday activities in ways positively influencing child learning and development. A lesson learned some 20 years ago (Dunst & Leet, 1987; Dunst, Leet, & Trivette, 1988) was the fact that family concerns unrelated to child rearing interfere with their willingness to implement practices as part of their involvement in early childhood intervention programs. For this reason, it is important to recognize that CMP is best understood in the context of a broader-based framework of family systems intervention.

ACKNOWLEDGMENTS

The preparation of this chapter was supported, in part, by Grant Nos. H324M010055, H024S960008, and H024B60119 funded by the U.S. Department of Education, Office of Special Education Programs, Research to Practice Division. The opinions expressed, however, are those of the authors and do not necessarily reflect the official position of the Department of Education.

REFERENCES

Alvarez, A. (1994). Child's everyday life: An ecological approach to the study of activity systems. In A. Alvarez & P. del Río (Eds.), *Educations as cultural construction* (Explorations in socio-cultural studies, pp. 23–38). Madrid, Spain: Fundación Infancia y Aprendizaje.

Bandura, A. (1997). *Self-efficacy: The exercise of control*. New York: Freeman.

Beckman, P., Barnwell, D., Horn, E., Hanson, M., Guitierrez, S., & Lieber, J. (1998). Communities, families and inclusion. *Early Childhood Research Quarterly, 13*, 125–150.

Bourdieu, P. (1977). *Outline of a theory of practice*. Cambridge, UK: Cambridge University Press.

Bronfenbrenner, U. (1979). *The ecology of human development: Experiments by nature and design*. Cambridge, MA: Harvard University Press.

Bronfenbrenner, U. (1992). Ecological systems theory. In R. Vasta (Ed.), *Six theories of child development: Revised formulations and current issues* (pp. 187–248). Philadelphia: Jessica Kingsley.

Bronfenbrenner, U. (1993). The ecology of cognitive development: Research models and fugitive findings. In R. H. Wozniak & K. W. Fischer (Eds.), *Development in context: Acting and thinking in specific environments* (pp. 3–44). Hillsdale, NJ: Erlbaum.

Bronfenbrenner, U. (1999). Environments in developmental perspective: Theoretical and operational models. In S. L. Friedman & T. D. Wachs (Eds.), *Measuring environment across the life span: Emerging methods and concepts* (pp. 3–28). Washington, DC: American Psychological Association.

Chaiklin, S., Hedegaard, M., & Jensen, U. J. (Eds.). (1999). *Activity theory and social practice: Cultural-historical approaches*. Aarhus C, Denmark: Aarhus University Press.

Chaiklin, S., & Lave, J. (Eds.). (1996). *Understanding practice: Perspectives on activity and context*. Cambridge, UK: Cambridge University Press.

Coleman, P. K., & Karraker, K. H. (2003). Maternal self-efficacy beliefs, competence in parenting, and toddlers' behavior and developmental status. *Infant Mental Health Journal, 24*, 126–148.

Coleman, P. K., Trent, A., Bryan, S., King, B., Rogers, N., & Nazir, M. (2002). Parenting behavior, mothers' self-efficacy beliefs, and toddler performance on the Bayley Scales of Infant Development. *Early Child Development and Care, 172*, 123–140.

Duchan, J. F. (1997). A situated pragmatics approach for supporting children with severe communication disorders. *Topics in Language Disorders, 17*(2), 1–18.

Dunst, C. J. (1979). Cognitive–social aspects of communicative exchanges between mothers and their Down's syndrome infants and mothers and their nonretarded infants. *Dissertation Abstracts International, 41*(01), 376B.

Dunst, C. J. (1981). *Infant learning: A cognitive–linguistic intervention strategy*. Allen, TX: DLM.

Dunst, C. J. (1985). Rethinking early intervention. *Analysis and Intervention in Developmental Disabilities, 5*, 165–201.

Dunst, C. J. (1992). A "new look" at promoting the development of children with Down syndrome. In P. Ryall (Ed.), *Learning together* (pp. 3–7). Calgary, Alberta, Canada: Canadian Down Syndrome Society.

Dunst, C. J. (2000). Everyday children's learning opportunities: Characteristics and consequences. *Children's Learning Opportunities Report, 2*(1). Available at *www.everydaylearning.info/reports/lov2-1.pdf*.

Dunst, C. J. (2001). Participation of young children with disabilities in community learning activities. In M. J. Guralnick (Ed.), *Early childhood inclusion: Focus on change* (pp. 307–333). Baltimore: Brookes.

Dunst, C. J. (2004). An integrated framework for practicing early childhood intervention and family support. *Perspectives in Education, 22*(2), 1–16.

Dunst, C. J. (2006). Parent-mediated everyday child learning opportunities: I. Foundations and operationalization. *CASEinPoint, 2*(2), 1–10. Available at *www.fippcase.org/caseinpoint/caseinpoint_vol2_no2.pdf*.

Dunst, C. J. (2007). Early intervention with infants and toddlers with developmental disabilities. In S. L. Odom, R. H. Horner, M. Snell, & J. Blacher (Eds.), *Handbook of developmental disabilities* (pp. 161–180). New York: Guilford Press.

Dunst, C. J., Brookfield, J., & Epstein, J. (1998, December). *Family-centered early intervention and child, parent and family benefits: Final report.* Asheville, NC: Orelena Hawks Puckett Institute.

Dunst, C. J., Bruder, M. B., Trivette, C. M., & Hamby, D. W. (2006). Everyday activity settings, natural learning environments, and early intervention practices. *Journal of Policy and Practice in Intellectual Disabilities, 3*, 3–10.

Dunst, C. J., Bruder, M. B., Trivette, C. M., Hamby, D., Raab, M., & McLean, M. (2001). Characteristics and consequences of everyday natural learning opportunities. *Topics in Early Childhood Special Education, 21*, 68–92.

Dunst, C. J., & Hamby, D. (1999a). Community life as sources of children's learning opportunities. *Children's Learning Opportunities Report, 1*(4). Available at *www.everydaylearning.info/reports/lov1-4.pdf*.

Dunst, C. J., & Hamby, D. (1999b). Family life as sources of children's learning opportunities. *Children's Learning Opportunities Report, 1*(3). Available at *www.everydaylearning.info/reports/lov1-3.pdf*.

Dunst, C. J., Hamby, D., Trivette, C. M., Raab, M., & Bruder, M. B. (2000). Everyday family and community life and children's naturally occurring learning opportunities. *Journal of Early Intervention, 23*, 151–164.

Dunst, C. J., Hamby, D., Trivette, C. M., Raab, M., & Bruder, M. B. (2002). Young children's participation in everyday family and community activity. *Psychological Reports, 91*, 875–897.

Dunst, C. J., Hamby, D. W., & Brookfield, J. (2007). Modeling the effects of early childhood intervention variables on parent and family well-being. *Journal of Applied Quantitative Methods, 2*, 268–288.

Dunst, C. J., Holbert, K. A., & Wilson, L. L. (1990). Strategies for assessing infant sensorimotor interactive competencies. In E. Gibbs & D. Teti (Eds.), *Interdisciplinary assessment of infants: A guide for early intervention practitioners* (pp. 91–112). Baltimore: Brookes.

Dunst, C. J., & Kassow, D. Z. (2008). Caregiver sensitivity, contingent social responsiveness, and secure infant attachment. *Journal of Early and Intensive Behavior Intervention, 5*, 40–56.

Dunst, C. J., & Leet, H. E. (1987). Measuring the adequacy of resources in households with young children. *Child: Care, Health and Development, 13*, 111–125.

Dunst, C. J., Leet, H. E., & Trivette, C. M. (1988). Family resources, personal well-being, and early intervention. *Journal of Special Education, 22*, 108–116.

Dunst, C. J., Lesko, J. J., Holbert, K. A., Wilson, L. L., Sharpe, K. L., & Ritchie, F. L. (1987). A systemic approach to infant intervention. *Topics in Early Childhood Special Education, 7*(2), 19–37.

Dunst, C. J., Lowe, L. W., & Bartholomew, P. C. (1990). Contingent social responsiveness, family ecology, and infant communicative competence. *NSSLHA Journal, 17*, 39–49.

Dunst, C. J., & McWilliam, R. A. (1988). Cognitive assessment of multiply handicapped young children. In T. D. Wachs & R. Sheehan (Eds.), *Assessment of young developmentally disabled children* (pp. 213–238). New York: Plenum Press.

Dunst, C. J., Pace, J., & Hamby, D. W. (2007). *Evaluation of the games for growing tool kit for promoting early contingency learning* (Winterberry Research Perspectives Vol. 1, No. 6). Asheville, NC: Winterberry Press.

Dunst, C. J., & Raab, M. (2004). Parents' and practitioners' perspectives of young children's everyday natural learning environments. *Psychological Reports, 93,* 251–256.

Dunst, C. J., Raab, M., Trivette, C. M., Parkey, C., Gatens, M., Wilson, L. L., et al. (2007). Child and adult social–emotional benefits of response-contingent child learning opportunities. *Journal of Early and Intensive Behavior Intervention, 4,* 379–391.

Dunst, C. J., & Shue, P. (2005). Creating literacy-rich natural learning environments for infants, toddlers, and preschoolers. In E. M. Horn & H. Jones (Eds.), *Supporting early literacy development in young children* (Young Exceptional Children Monograph Series No. 7, pp. 15–30). Longmont, CO: Sopris West.

Dunst, C. J., & Swanson, J. (2006). Parent-mediated everyday child learning opportunities: II. Methods and procedures. *CASEinPoint, 2*(11), 1–19. Available at *www.fippcase.org/caseinpoint/caseinpoint_vol2_no11.pdf*.

Dunst, C. J., & Trivette, C. M. (2003). *Child learning opportunities scale.* Asheville, NC: Winterberry Press.

Dunst, C. J., & Trivette, C. M. (2009). Capacity-building family-systems intervention practices. *Journal of Family Social Work, 12* 119–143.

Dunst, C. J., Trivette, C. M., & Cutspec, P. A. (2007). *An evidence-based approach to documenting the characteristics and consequences of early intervention practices* (Winterberry Research Perspectives Vol. 1, No. 2). Asheville, NC: Winterberry Press.

Dunst, C. J., Trivette, C. M., & Hamby, D. W. (2006). *Family support program quality and parent, family and child benefits* (Winterberry Monograph Series). Asheville, NC: Winterberry Press.

Dunst, C. J., Trivette, C. M., & Hamby, D. W. (2008). *Research synthesis and meta-analysis of studies of family-centered practices* (Winterberry Monograph Series). Asheville, NC: Winterberry Press.

Dunst, C. J., Trivette, C. M., Hamby, D. W., & Bruder, M. B. (2006). Influences of contrasting natural learning environment experiences on child, parent, and family well-being. *Journal of Developmental and Physical Disabilities, 18,* 235–250.

Dunst, C. J., Trivette, C. M., Humphries, T., Raab, M., & Roper, N. (2001). Contrasting approaches to natural learning environment interventions. *Infants and Young Children, 14*(2), 48–63.

Ehrmann, L. C., Aeschleman, S. R., & Svanum, S. (1995). Parental reports of community activity patterns: A comparison between young children with disabilities and their nondisabled peers. *Research in Developmental Disabilities, 16,* 331–343.

Farver, J. A. M. (1999). Activity setting analysis: A model for examining the role of culture in development. In A. Göncü (Ed.), *Children's engagement in the world: Sociocultural perspectives* (pp. 99–127). Cambridge, UK: Cambridge University Press.

Fogel, A. (1997). Information, creativity, and culture. In C. Dent-Read & P. Zukow-Goldring (Eds.), *Evolving explanations of development: Ecological approaches to organism–environment systems* (pp. 413–443). Washington, DC: American Psychological Association.

Gallimore, R., Goldenberg, C. N., & Weisner, T. S. (1993). The social construction and subjective reality of activity settings: Implications for community psychology. *American Journal of Community Psychology, 21*, 537–559.

Gallimore, R., Weisner, T. S., Bernheimer, L. P., Guthrie, D., & Nihira, K. (1993). Family responses to young children with developmental delays: Accommodation activity in ecological and cultural context. *American Journal on Mental Retardation, 98*, 185–206.

Gallimore, R., Weisner, T. S., Kaufman, S. Z., & Bernheimer, L. P. (1989). The social construction of ecocultural niches: Family accommodation of developmentally delayed children. *American Journal on Mental Retardation, 94*, 216–230.

Goldberg, S. (1977). Social competence in infancy: A model of parent–infant interaction. *Merrill–Palmer Quarterly, 23*, 163–177.

Göncü, A. (Ed.). (1999). *Children's engagement in the world: Sociocultural perspectives*. Cambridge, UK: Cambridge University Press.

Göncü, A., Tuermer, U., Jain, J., & Johnson, D. (1999). Children's play as cultural activity. In A. Göncü (Ed.), *Children's engagement in the world: Sociocultural perspectives* (pp. 148–170). Cambridge, UK: Cambridge University Press.

Guberman, S. R. (1999). Supportive environments for cognitive development: Illustrations from children's mathematical activities outside of school. In A. Göncü (Ed.), *Children's engagement in the world: Sociocultural perspectives* (pp. 202–227). Cambridge, UK: Cambridge University Press.

Hatcher, B., & Beck, S. S. (Eds.). (1997). *Learning opportunities beyond the school* (2nd ed.). Olney, MD: Association for Childhood Education International.

Hewlett, S. A., & West, C. (1998). *The war against parents: What we can do for America's beleaguered moms and dads*. Boston: Houghton Mifflin.

Janes, H., & Kermani, H. (2001). Caregivers' story reading to young children in family literacy programs: Pleasure or punishment? *Journal of Adolescent and Adult Literacy, 44*, 458–466.

Kassow, D. Z., & Dunst, C. J. (2007a). *Characteristics of parental sensitivity related to secure infant attachment* (Winterberry Research Syntheses Vol. 1, No. 23). Asheville, NC: Winterberry Press.

Kassow, D. Z., & Dunst, C. J. (2007b). *Relationship between parental contingent-responsiveness and attachment outcomes* (Winterberry Research Syntheses Vol. 1, No. 1). Asheville, NC: Winterberry Press.

Krapp, A., Hidi, S., & Renninger, K. (1992). Interest, learning and development. In K. Renninger, S. Hidi, & A. Krapp (Eds.), *The role of interest in learning and development* (pp. 3–25). Hillsdale, NJ: Erlbaum.

Lamb, M. E., Leyendecker, B., Schölmerich, A., & Fracasso, M. P. (1998). Everyday experiences of infants in Euro-American and Central American immigrant families. In M. Lewis & C. Feiring (Eds.), *Families, risk, and competence* (pp. 113–131). Mahwah, NJ: Erlbaum.

Lancy, D. F. (1996). *Playing on the mother-ground: Cultural routines for children's development*. New York: Guilford Press.

Lave, J. (1996). The practice of learning. In S. Chaiklin & J. Lave (Eds.), *Understanding practice: Perspectives on activity and context* (pp. 3–32). Cambridge, UK: Cambridge University Press.

Lave, J., & Wenger, E. (1991). *Situated learning: Legitimate peripheral participation*. New York: Cambridge University Press.

MacTurk, R. H., & Morgan, G. A. (Eds.). (1995). *Mastery motivation: Origins, conceptualizations, and applications* (Advances in Applied Developmental Psychology Vol. 12). Norwood, NJ: Ablex.

McWilliam, R. A. (2000). It's only natural . . . to have early intervention in the environments where it's needed. In S. Sandall & M. Ostrosky (Eds.), *Natural environments and inclusion* (Young Exceptional Children Monograph Series No. 2, pp. 17–26). Longmont, CO: Sopris West.

McWilliam, R. A., & Ware, W. B. (1994). The reliability of observations of young children's engagement: An application of generalizability theory. *Journal of Early Intervention, 18,* 34–47.

Nelson, K. (1999, Winter). Making sense: Language and thought in development. *Developmental Psychologist,* 1–10.

Nievar, M. A., & Becker, B. J. (2008). Sensitivity as a privileged predictor of attachment: A second perspective on De Wolff and van IJzendoorn's meta-analysis. *Social Development, 17,* 102–114.

Okagaki, L., & Divecha, D. J. (1993). Development of parental beliefs. In T. Luster & L. Okagaki (Eds.), *Parenting: An ecological perspective* (pp. 35–67). Hillsdale, NJ: Erlbaum.

Raab, M. (2005). Interest-based child participation in everyday learning activities. *CASEinPoint, 1*(2), 1–5. Available at *www.fippcase.org/caseinpoint/caseinpoint_vol1_no2.pdf.*

Raab, M., & Dunst, C. J. (2004). Early intervention practitioner approaches to natural environment interventions. *Journal of Early Intervention, 27,* 15–26.

Raab, M., & Dunst, C. J. (2007). *Influence of child interests on variations in child behavior and functioning* (Winterberry Research Syntheses Vol. 1, No. 21). Asheville, NC: Winterberry Press.

Renninger, K. A. (1998). The roles of individual interest(s) and gender in learning: An overview of research on preschool and elementary school-aged children/students. In L. Hoffman, A. Krapp, K. A. Renninger, & J. Baumert (Eds.), *Interest and learning: Proceedings of the Seeon Conference on Interest and Gender* (pp. 165–174). Kiel, Germany: IPN.

Renninger, K. A., Hidi, S., & Krapp, A. (Eds.). (1992). *The role of interests in learning and development.* Hillsdale, NJ: Erlbaum.

Rogoff, B., Mosier, C., Mistry, J., & Göncü, A. (1993). Toddlers' guided participation with their caregivers in cultural activity. In E. A. Forman, N. Minick, & C. A. Stone (Eds.), *Contexts for learning: Sociocultural dynamics in children's development* (pp. 230–253). New York: Oxford University Press.

Rusher, A. S., Cross, D. R., & Ware, A. M. (1995). Infant and toddler play: Assessment of exploratory style and development level. *Early Childhood Research Quarterly, 10,* 297–315.

Shonkoff, J. P., & Phillips, D. A. (Eds.). (2000). *From neurons to neighborhoods: The science of early childhood development.* Washington, DC: National Academy Press.

Shweder, R. A., Goodnow, J., Hatano, G., LeVine, R. A., Markus, H., & Miller, P. (1998). The cultural psychology of development: One mind, many mentalities. In W. Damon & R. M. Lerner (Eds.), *Handbook of child psychology: Vol. 1. Theoretical models of human development* (5th ed., pp. 865–937). New York: Wiley.

Teti, D. M., & Gelfand, D. M. (1991). Behavioral competence among mothers of infants in the first year: The mediational role of maternal self-efficacy. *Child Development, 62,* 918–929.

Tharp, R., & Gallimore, R. (1988). *Rousing minds to life: Teaching, learning, and schooling in social context*. Cambridge, UK: Cambridge University Press.

Trevarthen, C., & Hubley, P. (1978). Secondary intersubjectivity: Confidence, confiding and acts of meaning in the first year. In A. Lock (Ed.), *Action, gesture, and symbol: The emergence of language* (pp. 183–232). New York: Academic Press.

Trivette, C. M. (2007). *Influence of caregiver responsiveness on the development of young children with or at risk for developmental disabilities* (Winterberry Research Syntheses Vol. 1, No. 12). Asheville, NC: Winterberry Press.

Trivette, C. M., Dunst, C. J., & Hamby, D. (2004). Sources of variation in and consequences of everyday activity settings on child and parenting functioning. *Perspectives in Education, 22*(2), 17–35.

Trivette, C. M., Dunst, C. J., Hamby, D. W., & Pace, J. (2007). *Evaluation of the tune in and respond tool kit for promoting child cognitive and social–emotional development* (Winterberry Research Perspectives Vol. 1, No. 7). Asheville, NC: Winterberry Press.

Tudge, J., Hogan, D., Lee, S., Tammeveski, P., Meltsas, M., Kulakova, N., et al. (1999). Cultural heterogeneity: Parental values and beliefs and their preschoolers' activities in the United States, South Korea, Russia, and Estonia. In A. Göncü (Ed.), *Children's engagement in the world: Sociocultural perspectives* (pp. 62–96). Cambridge, UK: Cambridge University Press.

Wachs, T. D. (1979). Proximal experience and early cognitive–intellectual development: The physical environment. *Merrill–Palmer Quarterly, 25*, 3–41.

Wachs, T. D. (2000). *Necessary but not sufficient: The respective roles of single and multiple influences on individual development*. Washington, DC: American Psychological Association.

Child Interests Checklist

This checklist includes a series of questions a practitioner can use to help a parent or other primary caregiver identify a child's interests. Indicate *Yes* or *No* whether or not your interactions with a parent involved the use of each of the interest identification methods.

Did you the practitioner help the parent . . .	Yes	No
1. Identify the objects, people, activities, and actions that capture and hold the child's attention?		
2. Identify the objects, people, activities, and actions that are the child's favorites?		
3. Identify the objects, people, activities, and actions that make the child smile and laugh?		
4. Identify the objects, people, activities, and actions that make the child feel happy and get excited?		
5. Identify the objects, people, activities, and actions that the child prefers?		
6. Identify the objects, people, activities, and actions that the child chooses to do or be with most often?		
7. Identify the objects, people, activities, and actions that the child spends time doing and works hard at doing?		

Everyday Community Learning Activity Checklist

This checklist includes a series of questions a practitioner can use to help a parent or other primary caregiver select interest-based everyday community learning activities and decide which activities would be the best learning opportunities. Indicate *Yes* or *No* whether or not your interactions with a parent involved the use of each of the checklist practices.

Did you the practitioner help the parent . . .	Yes	No
1. Identify the community activities that are the child's everyday life experiences?		
2. Identify those community activities that do or could provide the child interest-based learning opportunities?		
3. Identify interest-based community activities that happen occasionally, seasonally, or occur on special occasions?		
4. Select interest-based community activities that provide many different kinds of interest-based learning opportunities?		
5. Select interest-based community learning activities that do or could happen often?		
6. Select interest-based community learning activities where each activity provides lots of different learning opportunities?		
7. Select interest-based community learning activities that are especially likely to help the child practice emerging abilities and develop new ones?		
8. Select interest-based community activities that allow the child to try to do lots of different things?		

Increasing Everyday Child Learning Opportunities Checklist

This checklist includes a series of questions a practitioner can use to help a parent or other primary caregiver increase the *breadth* or *depth* of interest-based everyday child learning opportunities. Indicate *Yes* or *No* whether or not your interactions with a parent involved the use of each of the practices.		
Did you the practitioner help the parent . . .	Yes	No
1. Use a reminder list, calendar, or other kind of activity schedule to *increase how often* the child participates in interest-based community learning activities?		
2. Increase the *number* of interest-based community child learning activities?		
3. Increase the *variety* of interest-based community child learning activities?		
4. Increase the *quality* of interest-based community child learning activities?		
5. Increase the *number* of child learning opportunities available *within* any one community activity?		
6. Increase the *variety* of child learning opportunities available *within* any one community activity?		
7. Increase the *quality* of child learning opportunities available *within* any one community activity?		
8. Increase participation in those activities that occur frequently enough to provide lots of child learning opportunities?		

Caregiver Responsive Teaching Checklist

This checklist includes a series of questions a practitioner can use to help a parent or other primary caregiver understand and use different interactional behaviors supporting and encouraging child learning and competence in interest-based everyday activities. Indicate *Yes* or *No* whether or not your interactions with a parent involved the parents' use of the practices.

Did you the practitioner help the parent . . .	Yes	No
1. Engage the child in interest-based community learning activities?		
2. Provide the child time to initiate interactions with people or objects in the activities?		
3. Pay attention to and notice when and how the child interacts with people and objects in the community activities?		
4. Respond promptly and positively to the child's interactions in ways that match the amount, pace, and intent of the child's behavior?		
5. Respond to the child's behavior with comments, joint interaction, gestures, and so forth to support child engagement in the activity?		
6. Respond to the child in ways that encourage the child to use his/her behavior in new and different ways?		
7. Add new materials or arrange the environment to encourage the child to use his/her interests to do something new or different?		
8. Encourage the child to use behaviors that are increasingly more complex?		
9. Provide the child many opportunities to use and practice newly learned behaviors in the community activities?		

Parent-Mediated Child Learning Evaluation Checklist

This checklist includes a series of questions a practitioner can use to help a parent or other primary caregiver evaluate the benefits of his or her efforts to provide a child interest-based everyday learning opportunities. Indicate *Yes* or *No* whether or not your interactions with a parent involved the parents' judgments of the benefits of everyday child learning.

Did you the practitioner help the parent . . .	Yes	No
1. Determine if the child had the opportunity to participate in many different community activities?		
2. Determine if the child had chances to do different things in any one community activity?		
3. Determine if the child initiated more interactions with people and objects in the community activities?		
4. Determine if the child displayed a greater variety of behaviors in the community activities?		
5. Determine whether the child initiated more complex interactions with people and objects in the community activities?		
6. Determine whether the child smiled, laughed, or showed enjoyment in response to his/her accomplishments during community activities?		
7. Determine those parenting behaviors that supported and encouraged child learning in the community activities?		
8. Determine which aspects of the provision of interest-based child learning opportunities were most gratifying to the parent?		
9. Recognize the important role the parent had in providing the child interest-based learning opportunities?		
10. Use the evaluative information to change the community activities used for interest-based learning?		

CHAPTER 4

Coordinating Services with Families

MARY BETH BRUDER

In 1986, Part H (now Part C) of the Individuals with Disabilities Education Act (IDEA) created a statewide early intervention program available to eligible infants, toddlers, and their families. The components of the program are complex and require a commitment to a number of philosophical beliefs and programmatic features such as family-centered care, cultural competence, team process, natural learning environments, and interagency collaboration (Dunst, 2007; Hanson & Bruder, 2001). By far, the most challenging of these components is collaboration: Families, early interventionists, and other providers must plan, implement, and evaluate early intervention services and supports through the development of an individualized family service plan (IFSP) for each eligible child and family. The plan's purpose is to document the process by which an eligible child will receive what he or she needs to achieve agreed-upon outcomes and the supports a family will receive to be able to meet the special needs of their child. This component is most challenging, in part because agencies, providers, and families, as they attempt collaboratively to individualize services and supports for an eligible child, have inherent complexities (Bruder & Bologna, 1993). Most recently, an added complexity to early intervention has been the congressional mandate for accountability of the Part C program through the collection of family and child outcomes (see *www. the-eco-center.org*).

One programmatic feature to assist in the collaborative components of statewide early intervention systems is the appointment of a service coordinator for each eligible child and family. This person is responsible for overseeing all the

TABLE 4.1. Service Coordinator Responsibilities

- Coordinate and implement evaluations and assessments.
- Facilitate and participate in the development, review, and evaluation of the IFSP.
- Assist family in identifying available service providers.
- Coordinate and monitor the delivery of available services.
- Inform families of the availability of advocacy services.
- Coordinate with medical and health providers.
- Facilitate the development of a transition plan to preschool services.

collaborative requirements of service delivery. Service coordination is defined by Part C as assisting and enabling the eligible child and his or her family to receive the rights, procedural safeguards, and services authorized to be provided under the state's early intervention program. This function includes coordinating all services across agency lines and serving as the single point of contact to help families obtain the services and assistance they need. To be qualified to do this, service coordinators must demonstrate knowledge and understanding about eligible infants and toddlers, Part C of IDEA and its regulations, the nature and scope of services available under a state early intervention system, and the payment system and other information. Within the law, seven specific activities are the responsibility of service coordinators; these include the development, monitoring, and implementation of a child and family's IFSP and ensuring ongoing coordination with other agencies and individuals providing services to the child and family. Table 4.1 lists these activities. The remainder of this chapter addresses these specific service coordination activities in depth, after first describing research that has contributed to a deeper understanding of the function and subsequent evaluation of service coordination under Part C of IDEA.

THE RESEARCH FOUNDATION FOR SERVICE COORDINATION

The Research and Training Center (RTC) on Service Coordination was funded by the Office of Special Education Programs (OSEP), U.S. Department of Education, to develop a model for training service coordinators under IDEA. To do this, a number of studies were conducted to identify the reality of service coordination across the country (Bruder & Dunst, 2006). Unfortunately, findings suggest that service coordination is not implemented consistently across the country (Harbin, et al, 2004). Nor is training of service coordinators required in the majority of states, and when required, the average length of training is 2.9 days (Bruder, 2005).

The RTC also conducted a second series of studies that sought to identify both the outcomes and practices of effective service coordination (Bruder et al., 2005; Dunst & Bruder, 2002, 2006). Through the use of multiple quantitative and qualitative methods of data collection, analysis, and synthesis, a series of national studies occurred. The breadth of the findings of the studies underscored the complexity of service coordination. For example, initially, over 250 service coordination outcomes and over 2,000 discrete practices were identified by participants in the studies. These data required extensive synthesis before a convergence of the multiple data sources resulted in nine interrelated outcomes that should be achieved as a result of high-quality service coordination (see Table 4.2), and three practice categories. The categories were helpgiving, collaboration, and administration.

To integrate these data on service coordination models, outcomes, and practices, the RTC adopted the ecological framework set forth by Bronfenbrenner (1993). This orientation requires attention to be given to the multiple characteristics of a service system, suggesting that child and family outcomes of service coordination are influenced by the individuals, organizations, agencies, cultures, communities, and states involved in service delivery and system administration. In addition, the child and family exist within a series of complex contexts such as their history, values, culture, ethnicity, structure, home routines and community activities, child disability, child age, economic status, and geographic location. Likewise, service providers and coordinators possess attitudes, values, knowledge (of resources and recommended practices), previous experiences, training, and skills that they bring to the service implementation endeavor. These characteristics of both the family and service provider also influence the multiple elements of service coordination. Lastly, service coordination is also influenced by the existing system infrastructure. The infrastructure is made up of multiple organizations, agencies, and programs that can facilitate or hinder effective service coordination. Although funding is an important piece of the infrastructure, other aspects of the infrastructure are equally important (e.g., personnel development, service coordination caseload policies).

Whereas the interrelationships among these variables describe the complexity of service coordination, they also challenge any model for training and evaluation. One such model designed for this type of a system is a logic model. A logic model

TABLE 4.2. Service Coordination Outcomes

- Families have access to support, information, and education to address their individual needs.
- Families are able to communicate the needs of their child.
- Families make informed decisions about services, resources, and opportunities for their child.
- Agencies and professionals are coordinated.
- Children and families receive quality service.
- Children and families participate in supports and services that are coordinated, effective, and individualized to their needs.
- Families acquire and/or maintain a quality of life to enhance their well-being.
- Families meet the special needs of their child.
- Children's health and development are enhanced.

can be used to create an understanding of the interrelationships of variables that contribute to a program or program feature (e.g., service coordination). Variables can be grouped according to characteristics such as resources or inputs, activities, outputs, and outcomes (Gilliam & Mayes, 2000; W. K. Kellogg Foundation, 2001). Using the data described above, the RTC developed a logic model to show how service coordination should work. This model can guide the implementation and evaluation of service coordination for early intervention as in Figure 4.1. The test of the actual effectiveness of service coordination is how well the service coordinator implements the activities he or she is responsible for, as measured by a family, child, and system status in each of the outcomes presented in the logic model. The identified practice areas must be used in each of the discrete activities, and these will each be described. Checklists for these practices to be used for each activity are in the appendices at the end of this chapter.

COORDINATING THE PERFORMANCE OF EVALUATIONS AND ASSESSMENTS

The service coordinator serves as the single point of contact for families when they first enter the early intervention system. At this stage, families face the unknown. Some families may have never heard of early intervention, and others may not realize that their child has developmental needs. It is the service coordinator's responsibility to take the time to develop a relationship with the family, learn about their needs and concerns, and explain the early intervention system. These steps are critical to coordinating the initial evaluation and assessment to determine a child's eligibility for early intervention.

The initial contact and intake is the first step in coordinating evaluations and assessments. It should be in person and may involve more than one meeting, over time. Taking this time enables the service coordinator to build a relationship with the family and to learn about the child's and family's needs. Accomplishing these tasks requires the service coordinator to use helpgiving practices such as treating families with dignity and respect; to be culturally and socioeconomically sensitive to family diversity; to provide choices to families in relation to their priorities and concerns; to disclose information to families so they can make decisions; and to employ communication strategies to empower and enhance a family's competence and confidence (see Dunst, Trivette, & Handy, 2007). If done effectively, the evaluation and assessment process identifies child and family needs as well as the services and supports that will meet those needs. It is critical that service coordinators approach the evaluation and assessment process in ways that are respectful and sensitive to the family's needs and concerns and that they ensure that the family fully understands the evaluation process.

Because the service coordinator is responsible for arranging and coordinating the evaluations and assessments to determine a child's eligibility and need

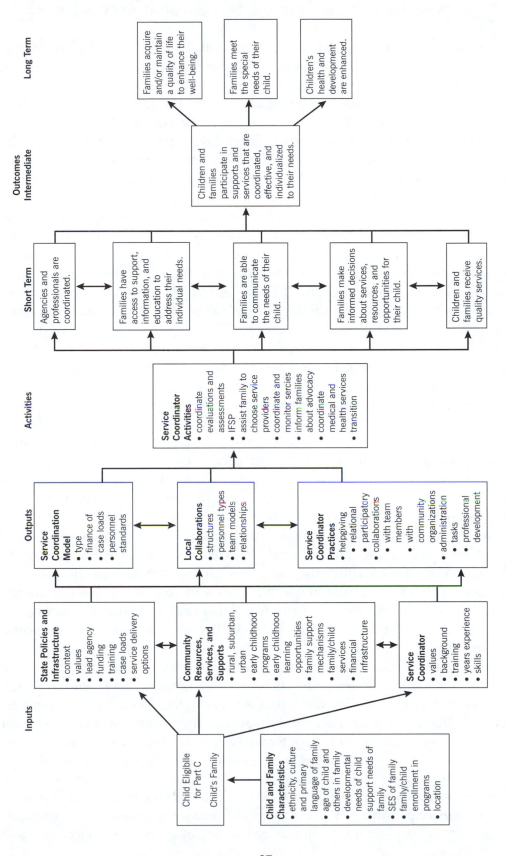

FIGURE 4.1. A logic model for service coordination.

97

for early intervention, before anything is done to the child, it is also his or her responsibility to ensure that the family is informed of their rights and procedural safeguards concerning participation in early intervention. Only then can the service coordinator begin to coordinate the actual implementation of evaluation and assessments. This coordination encompasses both the people who administer the assessment and the tools and processes used during the assessment. To qualify for services, most children will require an evaluation to determine eligibility. This assessment can serve a diagnostic function and create an accurate portrayal of the child's needs across medical, educational, and social systems. It should be noted that an eligibility assessment is not needed for children who may qualify for early intervention because they have received a diagnosis of a medical condition that qualifies as an established condition. A strong recommendation with regard to the diagnostic assessment is to focus on the process as opposed to just the product of the assessment. This practice supports the belief that it is extremely nonproductive to assess a very young child on developmental skills assigned by domain, because these domains are interdependent. Although IDEA requires that the current level of functioning of the child be reported by five domains, traditional assessment models (e.g., discipline specific, in a novel setting with contrived activities, conducted by strangers) prove inadequate when working with infants and toddlers with disabilities. Effective early childhood assessment protocols must rely on a sensitivity to the age of the child, the nature of the delay or disability, the family context, and the integration of a child's behaviors across developmental domains. This does not mean that professionals with discipline-specific expertise are not an important component of the assessment protocol, but, rather, they collaborate as a team on the assessment process and integrated assessment report, so that the child is seen as a whole, rather than domain by domain.

The service coordinator must ensure that a collaborative team process occurs before (planning), during (process), and after (reporting) an assessment. The service coordinator must identify the team members for the assessment and must develop a collaborative climate in which all can work together to obtain information about the child's development and functional abilities within the family and their community. The first challenge is to identify team members who are competent in both their discipline and in early development as well as team process and collaborative consultation. Although such competence has been advocated for many years in early intervention (cf., Bruder, 1996; Rapport, McWilliam, & Smith, 2004), evidence of the use of best practices is sparse (DEC, 1993). Nonetheless, Part C requires the use of multidisciplinary teams in the evaluation and assessment processes. The composition of these teams is then dictated by the unique needs of the child and family in relation to the purpose of assessment. For example, a diagnostic assessment may require more in-depth involvement from numerous professionals from a variety of specialized disciplines. If the objective is to present a comprehensive picture of the child's level of functioning across the five domains as required by law—motor, communication, social–emotional, cognition, and adaptive—numerous professionals might be involved. By law, two or more must be involved for it to constitute a multidisciplinary assessment.

A functional assessment for IFSP planning can also determine the child's current level of development, but it *focuses* on the child's participation in appropriate family and community activities and routines. It may be easier to accomplish this with fewer professionals because this assessment should either occur in the places where a child typically participates or in an interview format; too many people will be cumbersome at best and overwhelming at worst. The extent to which the child participates in these activities or routines (e.g., how often the child uses a spoon during meal times), using skills from all developmental domains, is the objective of this type of assessment, as opposed to the checking off of domain-specific skills. This type of assessment should also identify adaptations, supports, and strategies to increase the child's participation and learning in those activities or routines (e.g., spoons with built-up handles). The result is a complete and accurate picture of the child's current abilities and ability to learn in a variety of activities or routines. The child's competencies and strengths, preferences, and interests should be identified because parents and professionals can use these throughout the assessment. The assessment should engage the child in interesting activities to ensure that the child's performance is maximized. A functional assessment also focuses on observations of the way the social and physical environment helps or hinders the child's functioning within a specific activity or routine to identify adaptations to the environment that might facilitate child competence and participation.

Last, an integrated assessment report should be developed by the team for both an eligibility evaluation or comprehensive assessment for program planning. Assessment information must be summarized from the recorded observations, interviews, checklists, and scales. The purpose of the assessment report is to provide a picture of the child and his or her family to help create objectives and intervention adaptations, supports, and strategies. The report should be representative of the total process and should report child and family strengths as well as needs. A further suggestion would be for the service coordinator to conduct a routines-based interview with the family to maximize the impact of the developmental assessments to be done with the child (see R. A. McWilliam, Chapter 2, this volume).

DEVELOPMENT, REVIEW, AND EVALUATION OF THE IFSP

The service coordinator facilitates all aspects of the development, ongoing review, and annual evaluation of the IFSP. During each of these steps, the service coordinator is responsible for ensuring that everyone who is connected to the child—family, early intervention service providers, and community resources—come together to share their information and assessment results, develop child and family outcomes, and identify the services and supports needed to meet the IFSP outcomes. The IFSP is a working document, and the service coordinator is also responsible for ensuring that the plan reflects the child's and family's priorities and addresses any additional needs that arise. It should be written in family-friendly language, focus on the child's and family's strengths, and have measurable, obtainable outcomes and goals. The IFSP must also be comprehensive and collaborative if it is going to result in positive outcomes for a child and family. The collaborative components include integrated outcomes and objectives that cross discipline and agency boundaries, including coordination of social, medical, and health needs. The recommended interventions or services must be implemented within a child's natural environment, defined as those places where the child would be if he or she did not have disabilities.

An early intervention framework that provides a model for IFSP development is the use of family-identified activity settings and routines as the context of learning. These learning contexts support a variety of subcontexts that can be used to describe the experiences and learning opportunities given to children as part of daily living. They include child and family routines, family rituals, family and community celebrations, and family traditions. Most children, regardless of their disability or severity of delay, experience many kinds of learning opportunities daily, which should form the basis of ongoing therapeutic or instructional support. The IFSP outcomes should focus on facilitating the child's independent participation within and across activities and routines, as well as the expansion to additional learning opportunities across family- and provider-identified activity settings. The framework should be used by the service coordinator during both the assessment and the IFSP meeting.

The IFSP meeting brings service providers and the family together to engage in an exchange of information and joint decision making. Every IFSP team member contributes his or her knowledge to achieve a more in-depth understanding of the issues in supporting the child and the family. The initial IFSP meeting can set the tone for all IFSP meetings that follow. The service coordinator should use the following practices for effective and productive meetings.

Using Opening and Closing Activities

It can be helpful to begin a meeting with the opportunity for all team members to give information about themselves and their role in the IFSP process for that specific meeting. For example, an early interventionist may be the primary interventionist with one family, but with another family that person is a consultant to the primary interventionist who is directly involved in implementing the IFSP. By sharing this information, the team encourages discussion and creates a sense of equality among its members. This opportunity for sharing information among the team members is also important in helping the family to feel comfortable as they provide their perception of their role in the IFSP process.

Identifying the Team's Mission

A productive team has a clearly stated mission. A mission statement provides the team with a strong sense of purpose. In addition, a team is more likely to achieve its goals when it establishes a systematic work style, giving the team the organization and structure it needs to produce positive outcomes. The mission of an IFSP team should be focused on supporting the family members through the development of outcomes, objectives, and recommendations for interventions that meet their needs and interests. This goal should be clearly articulated at the beginning of the meeting by the service coordinator or a family member if he or she is interested.

Preparing an Agenda for Every Meeting

An agenda is an important tool for keeping a team focused on the same issues, and the service coordinator should develop one. A good agenda provides time for information exchange; discussion of specific task-related issues; and confirmation of the date, time, and place of the next meeting. By distributing the agenda before the day of the meeting, team members have the opportunity to prepare themselves for discussing agenda items.

Keeping Printed Minutes of Each Meeting

Minutes enhance team communication and should be taken at every meeting by the service coordinator. The team should select the member or members who will take and distribute minutes after each meeting. While there is no one standard format for minutes, they should include

- The names of the individuals who attended.
- The issues the meeting addressed.
- Any recommendations made.
- The team members responsible for implementing the recommendations.
- Timelines for completing follow-up tasks.

Preparing All Team Members for the Meeting

The experience with IFSP meetings may differ among team members. Unlike most of the early interventionists, family members and community service providers may have limited experience with IFSP meetings. An important task of the service coordinator is to help all team members prepare for the meeting by providing questions or issues to consider. This can help team members organize their thoughts ahead of time and facilitate their participation in discussion during the meeting.

After the family's concerns, priorities, resources, and activities and routines have been reviewed in the meeting, the next step is to translate this information into outcomes for the IFSP. Developing outcomes requires synthesizing available information and making decisions among competing priorities. It also requires negotiation, collaboration, and problem solving among team members, most importantly, the service coordinator. Although the family is the central focus of the process, team members who may have different perspectives or priorities should work together to negotiate values and priorities to reach a joint solution. The service coordinator should use and model effective communication strategies to help the team members, including the family, identify outcomes related to enhancing the development of the child.

Part C of IDEA specifies that the IFSP must include services needed to enhance the development of the child and the capacity of the family to meet the special needs of the child. To do this, IFSP outcomes should focus on the family as well as the child. Family outcomes are the changes family members want in their lives related to enhancing their child's development. Because each family is unique, the IFSP team should discuss the family's concerns, priorities, and resources, as well as activities and routines that the family desires to participate in as a family.

When writing family outcomes, it is important to include a statement of what is expected to occur or be accomplished. Moreover, family outcomes should be written in the family's language and easily understood. The Office of Special Education Programs (OSEP) in the U.S. Department of Education has recently identified three family outcome areas to be measured to assess families' progress in the Part C programs. The areas are a family's (1) knowing their rights, (2) being able to communicate their child's needs, and (3) being able to help their child learn and grow. Because these outcomes are broad and designed for accountability across large numbers of families, the service coordinator should assist the IFSP team to develop more relevant and specific outcomes with the family as needed. These could range from "The mother would like to find someone who she feels knows how to take care of Jack on Thursday nights so she can rejoin her church choir" to "The family would like to learn more about their child's disability and its implications for future development" to "The family would like to find a larger house that can accommodate the parents and three children." The first example focuses on the support the parent needs for child care and maintaining her social network. This outcome is also related to the child's development, because the parent feels that the support she gets from the church choir can help her reduce her stress. Decreasing stress and increasing support are important to the quality of caregiver–child relationships and interactions. In turn, positive caregiver–child relationships and interactions can contribute to positive child outcomes.

The second example focuses on the family's need for knowledge and information about their child's disability and how the disability can have an impact on the family's interactions with the child. Knowing the child's disability and development can help the family identify needed support and resources to take care of their child. The third example focuses on the family's need for alternative housing opportunities. Although this family outcome does not seem to be directly related to the child's development, it is actually important for the family because it is already living in a crowded apartment and would need additional space to accommodate their child with physical disabilities who is in a wheelchair. Being able to move around freely in the house is significant for the child to increase his or her independence and learning (e.g., reaching for toys and materials he or she wants, helping him- or herself with personal tasks). The service coordinator usually is responsible for coordinating the family as well as the child outcomes.

ASSISTING FAMILIES
IN CHOOSING AVAILABLE SERVICE PROVIDERS

No one in the field of early intervention would argue that infants and toddlers with disabilities or those at risk for disability often require the combined expertise of numerous personnel, services, and agencies. The identification of appropriately trained personnel to assist a child and family, however, can be challenging. When more than one type of service provider is needed, it can be almost impossible to identify providers who share an intervention philosophy and are willing to support the family as the target of the intervention. For example, personnel having medical expertise, therapeutic expertise, and educational/developmental and social services expertise traditionally have been involved in the provision of services to infants and young children with disabilities and their families. Each of these service providers might represent a different professional discipline, be employed by a different agency, and practice under conflicting philosophical models of service delivery. In fact, at the service level, coordination can be fraught with tension because of the inherent structure of personnel preparation programs and subsequent discipline-specific practices (Bruder & Dunst, 2005). Table 4.3 contains a listing and description of the most typical early intervention providers.

The additional concern about appropriately trained service providers was also identified by the Part C state coordinators. Forty-seven of them responded to a questionnaire in which they stated that the majority of their Part C workforce, across disciplines, were undertrained to provide early intervention. In fact, only 16 states require a credential specific to early intervention competencies for anyone providing services in their Part C system (for both studies, see *www.uconnucedd. org/per_prep_center/index.html*). As a result, assessing the availability and competence of service providers to assist the family to facilitate their child's development might be the service coordinator's most difficult task.

A service coordinator practice that can assist in this activity is the identification and use of a primary early intervention provider (chosen because he or she displays the competencies necessary to facilitate the child's development) who, through a relationship with the parent and other caregivers (including child care

TABLE 4.3. Professionals from Multiple Disciplines in Early Intervention

Discipline	Area of expertise
Speech–language pathologist	A speech–language pathologist focuses on a child's communication skills. He or she evaluates the quantity and quality of sounds a child makes and his or her communication strategies. A speech–language pathologist also determines whether there are physical problems that may interfere with a child's speech.
Early childhood special education teacher	An early childhood special education teacher focuses on a child's development across areas including social, self-help, behavior, movement, and language skills.
Occupational therapist	An occupational therapist focuses on a child's independence in carrying out daily living tasks (e.g., eating, dressing, toileting), and using fine motor skills. An occupational therapist evaluates a child's self-care skills, play manipulation skills, and other activities.
Physical therapist	A physical therapist focuses on a child's ability to move. Physical therapists have been trained to assess movement, muscle tone, muscle strengths, range of motion, and balance, as well as functional or pathological motor limitations.
Social worker	A social worker can provide counseling and direct a family to a broad range of community resources (e.g., church groups, private and public agencies, support groups). A social worker assesses a family's capacity to manage basic needs such as those for food, clothing, shelter, and medical care, as well as other support needs.
Psychologist	A psychologist assesses a family's and child's psychological status, such as the parents' stress level, coping skills, and the child's mental health.
Nutritionist	A nutritionist facilitates a child's development by ensuring he or she receives the quality and quantity of nutrients required to maintain health. A nutritionist assesses a child's food intake, and any feeding needs. The nutritionist can provide advice about diet and develop feeding care plans for the family.
Audiologist	An audiologist detects hearing problems and recommends procedures for managing a child's hearing loss. An audiologist is trained to conduct specialized evaluations that measure hearing.
Medical specialist	A medical specialist promotes a child's optimal health, growth, and development. A medical specialist is usually a doctor who diagnoses and treats health problems within his or her area of expertise.

providers), integrates recommendations from other discipline-specific providers when providing intervention to the child. A service coordinator can facilitate the family's comfort level with this model by using helpgiving skills such as providing information about providers who are competent to be a primary provider.

One necessary component of the primary provider model is the use of a transdisciplinary team because it focuses on the delivery of early intervention across developmental domains as opposed to having separate interventions delivered by professionals from different disciplines (King et al., 2009). The child's interventions are implemented by the primary early interventionist, with ongoing assistance provided by professionals from various disciplines. The additional team members serve as consultants to the primary early interventionist, as the primary provider serves as a consultant to the family and the community service providers. As a result, their abilities to facilitate the child's development and learning are enhanced. In deciding which professional in the team should be the primary early interventionist for an individual family, the service coordinator must consider a number of factors, including the following.

Family Interest and Child Characteristics

The competencies of the primary early interventionist should fit the family's interest and the child's characteristics, rather than the specific skills associated with a particular discipline. Other criteria for the primary early interventionist include an open and trusting relationship with the family, an understanding of the child's needs and the activity settings he or she participates in, and an ability to provide appropriate support to the community service providers.

The Skills and Knowledge of Individual Team Members

The primary early interventionist should have the skills to address functional development and participation within and across activity settings. In addition, the primary early interventionist should feel comfortable in his or her role as a consultant to the family. For example, a physical therapist may be selected as the primary early interventionist because he or she can provide recommendations related to a child's participation in the various activity settings available at a park, riding in a canoe, eating dinner, and taking a bath. When the child has needs in other developmental areas, the primary early interventionist should be able to attend to them as well.

The Availability of the Primary Early Interventionist

For families and community members to feel confident and competent, the primary early interventionist must provide consultation within the activities and routines where the intervention will be implemented. The primary early interventionist must also have the flexibility to participate in a variety of activities and routines, because families might feel uncomfortable generalizing the intervention to other settings where consultation has not yet occurred.

Some interventionists might have the competency to provide consultation on child participation across developmental domains but not have the ability to observe within and across all the activities and routines identified by the family. For example, a special educator who teaches in a classroom during the day and works as an early interventionist at night has been the EI consultant to a family during the activity setting of eating dinner. The family has questions, however, about implementing the intervention during breakfast, and the interventionist has not been able to observe the child when eating lunch at the child care program. Although the interventionist could ideally consult during breakfast on the weekend, this does not work for the child care program, which is only open weekdays. When determining who is best suited to be the primary early interventionist for a particular family, the availability of the interventionist must be considered.

Using a primary provider model and transdisciplinary team approach requires a high level of communication and collaboration among team members. The service coordinator must be able to assist the team to negotiate and problem solve. Additionally, the service coordinator must have an understanding of the professional training and expertise across all team members to facilitate role release, which is a process of teaching, sharing, and exchanging of certain roles and responsibilities among the team members. Role release allows the primary early interventionist to obtain support from other team members to carry out activities that would be normally the responsibility of other team members. In order to implement the process of role release effectively, team members must be willing to learn from the skills and expertise of other team members. Team members can learn the techniques of another discipline through activities such as asking a professional from another discipline for explanation of unfamiliar technical language or jargon; watching a professional from another discipline work with a child and discuss perceptions of what was observed; practicing a technique from another discipline and having a team member from that discipline critique that performance; working with a professional from another discipline side by side when implementing the intervention to a child; asking for help regarding the intervention; and discussing a child's performance with a professional from another discipline.

In addition, team members must be willing to share knowledge with other team members, such as suggesting adaptations or supports for a child to participate in activities and routines, recommending intervention strategies, and teaching the primary early interventionist how to support development and learning in all domains. Each team member, however, continues to be recognized as the authority of his or her own discipline. Assistance and support for this role release should be provided by the service coordinator.

COORDINATING AND MONITORING THE DELIVERY OF AVAILABLE SERVICES

A comprehensive program can only be effective if data are collected regularly on child and family service implementation, learning opportunities, intervention strategies, and developmental and behavioral outcomes. The service coordinator serves as the single point of contact in helping the family coordinate and monitor the provision of services and supports across disciplines and agency lines. It is the service coordinator's responsibility to ensure that all services and supports (1) are provided (or accessed) as outlined in the IFSP, (2) are delivered in a timely fashion and at times and places convenient to the family, (3) reflect current research concerning evidence-based practices, (4) are coordinated with one another, and (5) are continuously evaluated for their effectiveness. When service coordinators work to coordinate services and supports, they increase productivity and decrease stress for everyone involved. Quality service coordination ensures that everyone is working toward common goals, communicating openly, sharing effective intervention practices, and continually monitoring child and family status. As with other components, this approach requires a philosophy of coordination and integration, because services and outcomes should be measured only within a collaborative framework.

Examining child progress has two components. One is typically a part of IFSP reviews and ongoing data collection. Although snapshots of child and family progress are provided at regularly scheduled intervals, keeping track of progress continuously and across multiple activities and routines is critical to assessing whether the adaptations, supports, and intervention strategies have had an impact on the child and family.

One way to facilitate this service coordination activity is regular, scheduled team meetings in which professionals meet with the service coordinator and family to review and monitor a child's and family's progress through the early intervention service plan. Unfortunately, the reason these meetings don't occur with regularity is because of a lack of infrastructure supports such as funding for meeting times. However, both satisfaction and progress are reported in those systems where such meetings occur, and many professionals have recommended the use of such meetings to ensure ongoing collaboration and accountability. At a minimum, the IFSP biannual update meeting can be used to collect data for the federal report required of each state.

A second and more formal method of monitoring the delivery of early intervention is the annual performance reports required by OSEP for all Part C participants (see *www.the-eco-center.org*). The specific outcomes that are to be used for reporting are on Table 4.2. Unfortunately at this time, states are able to organize this Part C data collection specific to their state needs and current practices, thus creating challenges to the ultimate validity of the national effort. Nonetheless, states should avail themselves of the opportunity to design reliable and valid data systems for federal and state requirements.

INFORMING FAMILIES OF THE AVAILABILITY OF ADVOCACY SERVICES

Families, as a rule, know their children's needs best. Gaining access to the services to meet those needs means that families sometimes have to request, even demand, that those services be provided. An important function that service coordinators fulfill is helping families become strong advocates for their children. The term *advocacy* refers to speaking on behalf of others. Service coordinators help by informing families about advocacy services that are available to them: services that help families learn how to advocate, local and state services that can advocate on behalf of the individual family, and national organizations that advocate on behalf of children with special needs and their families in general. This is a critical activity for families who may want different, more, or fewer services than the IFSP team offers.

COORDINATING WITH MEDICAL AND HEALTH PROVIDERS

The coordination of early intervention with medical and health providers is an ongoing activity of early intervention. All children eligible for early intervention will have been seen by a health care provider prior to entry into early intervention. As the single point of contact for early intervention, service coordinators can help families improve coordination with their health care providers. Additionally, the service coordinator can help families obtain any additional medical and health providers families need and coordinate those services with other early intervention services and supports.

Many children who receive early intervention support have more than one medical and health provider. With multiple providers, care can easily become fragmented, and it is common for providers not to communicate or send reports to one another. This is one of the reasons the concept of a *medical home* has been advocated for all children, most importantly for children with special health care needs, many of whom will receive early intervention services. A medical home ensures that medical care is accessible to all children and coordinates all of a child's medical needs. A medical home can be a clinic, a primary care physician, or a group practice. The medical home is also responsible for ensuring the competence of all who provide services to a child and that financial resources are available for families to pay for necessary medical services. Last, the medical home also provides family supports that enable a family to meet the special needs of their child. Service coordinators should, therefore, identify a medical home for each child they serve, and ensure that information from the early intervention team is provided to the child's medical home.

Coordinating with medical and health providers also requires that the service coordinator obtain information from the medical home for the early intervention team. Early interventionists and other providers need health and medical information to determine how a child's health status affects not only overall development but also how it influences interventions with the child. Families must have up-to-date information on their child's health status to participate fully in their child's care. Finally, before any service providers can provide support for a child, they need information about a child's other needs and the services he or she already has.

FACILITATING THE DEVELOPMENT OF A TRANSITION PLAN TO PRESCHOOL SERVICES

The importance of transition has been addressed in state and federal legislation, federal funding initiatives, and the literature. A successful transition is a series of well-planned steps to facilitate the movement of the child and family into another setting (Bruder & Chandler, 1993). Coordinating successful transitions are a major responsibility of a service coordinator under Part C of IDEA. Needless to say, the type of planning and practices that are employed can influence the success of transition and satisfaction with the transition process.

Within the field of early intervention, transition is defined as the process of moving from one program to another or from one service delivery mode to another. Other people have emphasized the dynamic process of transition, as children with disabilities and their families will have repeated moves among different service providers, programs, and agencies as the child ages. Although formal transition for young children with disabilities typically occurs at age 3 (into preschool), transition between services, providers, and programs can also occur throughout these early years. Part C of IDEA increases the potential number of transitions. For example, transition can begin for some children at the moment of birth if it is determined that their health status requires transfer to a special care nursery and subsequent developmental interventions.

Children and families in early intervention might experience a number of transitions during the child's first 3 years of life. These transitions include moving from the hospital or neonatal intensive care unit to home; from home to various community settings; and, when the child turns 3 years old, to public school preschool or other community-based resources and supports. When families were asked about the most important outcomes for service coordination as part of our research, we found that successful transitions were a primary concern. Many families talked about how difficult this process can be and how an effective service coordinator will know the local school system and encourage families to visit different types of preschool programs. Well-developed transition plans should decrease additional assessments and paperwork and ensure that there are no time lags in service provision.

Many families do not realize that their child is not automatically eligible for services and supports after they exit the early intervention program. A good transition plan pulls together people and information so that everyone is well-informed and participates in the decision making. Successful transition plans provide families with knowledge and supports to obtain needed resources. Only when families are fully informed can they make decisions in partnership with other providers regarding future placement and services.

USING THE LOGIC MODEL TO FRAME EVALUATION

The implementation of service coordination activities may seem overwhelming, as they represent the process of early intervention for every eligible child and family. Therefore, the prospect of early intervention without a service coordinator is even more overwhelming. The attached checklists (Appendices 4.1–4.8) of practices for each activity are one means of accountability for the service coordinator, system, and family. The ultimate accountability focus, however, is the acquisition of service coordination outcomes as identified by the RTC (Table 4.2) for each eligible child and family.

As seen in Figure 4.1, the service coordination logic model has grouped the outcomes according to the immediacy of their acquisition. As with any logic model, operational measures must be used to address each one. The service coordinator should develop a series of measures that are applicable to each outcome for multiple points in the early intervention process. Interviews, checklists, and standard measures may be used together or alone, to address one outcome or all. These outcomes are embedded in the service coordination activities, practices, and state and local context, as displayed on the logic model. The measures used to document each outcome will ultimately allow an assessment of whether the intent of service coordination in Part C of IDEA is realized for families and their children.

CONCLUSION

Service coordination is the formation of all early intervention supports and services provided to infants, toddlers, and families. When done well, service coordination can be the light that illuminates the early intervention process for families. Likewise, service coordination can be the lynchpin to the use of evidence-based practices in early intervention for all service providers. When done poorly, however, service coordination adds to the complexity of early intervention by causing a negative impact on an already cumbersome system. This chapter provided some background research about and description of each of the seven activities of service coordination in an effort to provide practitioners and families the tools they need to implement service coordination effectively.

REFERENCES

Bronfenbrenner, U. (1993). The ecology of cognitive development: Research models and fugitive findings. In R. H. Wozniak & K. W. Fischer (Eds.), *Development in context: Acting and thinking in specific environments* (pp. 3–44). Hillsdale, NJ: Erlbaum.

Bruder, M. B. (1996). Interdisciplinary collaboration in service delivery. In R. A. McWilliam (Ed.), *Rethinking pull-out services in early intervention: A professional resource* (pp. 27–48). Fort Worth, TX: Harcourt Brace.

Bruder, M. B. (2005). Service coordination and integration in a developmental systems approach to early intervention. In M. J. Guralnick (Ed.), *A developmental systems approach to early intervention: National and international perspectives* (pp. 29–58). Baltimore: Brookes.

Bruder, M. B., & Bologna, T. M. (1993). Collaboration and service coordination for effective early intervention. In W. Brown, S. K. Thurman, & L. Pearl (Eds.), *Family-centered early intervention with infants and toddlers: Innovative cross-disciplinary approaches* (pp. 103–127). Baltimore: Brookes.

Bruder, M. B., & Chandler, L. K. (1993). Transition. In DEC (Ed.), *DEC recommended practices: Indicators of quality in programs for infants and young children with special needs and their families*. Reston, VA: Council for Exceptional Children.

Bruder, M. B., & Dunst, C. J. (2005). Personnel preparation in recommended early intervention practices: Degree of emphasis across disciplines. *Topics in Early Childhood Special Education, 25*(1), 25–33.

Bruder, M. B., & Dunst, C. J. (2006). Advancing the agenda of service coordination. *Journal of Early Intervention, 28*(3), 175–177.

Bruder, M. B., Harbin, G. L., Whitbread, K., Conn-Powers, M., Roberts, R., Dunst, C. J., et al. (2005). Establishing outcomes for service coordination: A step toward evidence-based practice. *Topics in Early Childhood Special Education, 25*(3), 177–188.

DEC. (Ed.). (1993). *DEC recommended practices: Indicators of quality in programs for infants and young children with special needs and their families*. Reston, VA: Council for Exceptional Children.

Dunst, C. J. (2007). Early intervention with infants and toddlers with developmental disabilities. In S. L. Odom, R. H. Horner, M. Snell, & J. Blacher (Eds.), *Handbook of developmental disabilities* (pp. 531–551). New York: Guilford Press.

Dunst, C. J., & Bruder, M. B. (2002). Valued outcomes of service coordination, early intervention and natural environments. *Exceptional Children, 68*(3), 361–375.

Dunst, C. J., & Bruder, M. B. (2006). Early intervention service coordination models and service coordinator practices. *Journal of Early Intervention, 28*(3), 155–165.

Gilliam, W. S., & Mayes, L. C. (2000). Development assessment of infants and toddlers. In C. H. Zeanah (Ed.), *Handbook of infant mental health* (2nd ed., pp. 236–248). New York: Guilford Press.

Hanson, M. J., & Bruder, M. B. (2001). Early intervention: Promises to keep. *Infants and Young Children, 13*(3), 47–58.

Harbin, G. L., Bruder, M. B., Whitbread, K., Reynolds, C., Mazzarella, C., Gabbard, G., et al. (2004). Early intervention service coordination policies: National policy infrastructure. *Topics in Early Childhood Special Education, 24*(2), 89–97.

King, G., Strachan, D., Tucker, M., Duwyn, B., Desserud, S., & Shillington, M. (2009) The application of a transdisciplinary model for early intervention services. *Infants and Young Children, 22*(3), 211–223.

Rapport, M. J. K., McWilliam, R. A., & Smith, B. J. (2004). Practices across disciplines in early intervention: The research base. *Infants and Young Children, 17*(1), 32–44.

W. K. Kellogg Foundation. (2001). *Using logic models to bring together planning, evaluation, and action: Logic model development guide*. Battle Creek, MI: Author.

Coordinating Evaluation and Assessments: First Contacts

The service coordinator will . . .	✓/✗	Notes
Share information about . . .		
• Early intervention (EI) philosophy		
• The statewide early intervention system including eligibility criteria for children		
• The difference between assessment for evaluation and ongoing assessment		
• The role of the family in the assessment process		
• Procedural safeguards and family rights		
• Confidentiality policies and practices		
Gather information from the family about . . .		
• Family background, ethnicity, and language preference		
• Family structure and composition		
• Child health and development status and history		
• Family resources, concerns, and priorities		
• Other agencies and professionals involved with the child		
• Their child's reaction to strangers (e.g., the interventionist)		
Collaborate to . . .		
• Identify methods of sharing information with others, including the family		

(cont.)

The service coordinator will . . .	✓/✗	Notes
Perform administrative tasks such as . . .		
• Get parent permission for the child's evaluation/assessment		
• Complete and submit to system releases for information		
• Complete and submit to system reimbursement information, if needed (e.g., insurance, Medicaid, family payment)		
• Get and share with the early intervention evaluators records and past assessments on the child		
• Gather information about the child's disability		
• Get parent permission to store data		
• Send a letter of acknowledgment about the family to the referral sources including the medical home		

Coordinating and Implementing Evaluations and Assessments

The service coordinator will . . .	✓/✗	Notes
Share information about . . .		
• Valid/reliable evaluation and assessment models and tools		
• The assessment protocol to be used		
• The family's role in the assessment		
• The assessment team and individual backgrounds of evaluators/assessors		
• The assessment tools to be used		
• Summary information on evaluation/assessment results		
Gather information from the family about . . .		
• The child and family activity settings/routines and the level of the child's participation within them		
• The child's typical behaviors, motivation, and persistence		
• Their preferred modality to receive the results summary of the evaluation/assessment		
• The child's reactions to new people		
• Adaptations and supports they use to facilitate their child's behavior		
Collaborate to . . .		
• Facilitate the sharing of information among team members (including the family) prior, during, and after the assessment		
• Assist the assessment team in the translation of evaluation/assessment results into functional applications within family-identified activity settings/routines		
• Assist the assessment team in writing up the assessment summary		

(cont.)

The service coordinator will . . .	✓/✗	Notes
Perform administrative tasks such as . . .		
• Identifying evaluation/assessment team members		
• Establishing evaluation/assessment time and place		
• Informing the family of the child's eligibility/non-eligibility for early intervention guidance about the next steps in the EI process		
• Providing guidance on child development services for children who do not quality for EI		

Facilitating and Participating in the Development, Review, and Evaluation of the IFSP

The service coordinator will . . .	✓/✗	Notes
Share information about . . .		
• The purpose of the IFSP		
• The IFSP meeting, format, and participants		
• The identification of EI services to enhance learning opportunities		
• The development of timelines and criteria for services		
• The evaluation criteria for service delivery and learning acquisition		
• The ongoing role of the service coordinator		
• The development of a transition plan		
Gather information from the family about . . .		
• Activity settings/routines for learning		
• Priorities for child participation in activity settings/routines		
• The identification of child learning opportunities in the home and community settings in which other children participate		
• The establishment of functional, integrated outcomes and objectives to support the child's and family's strengths in identified activity settings/routines		
• Time and place preferences for the IFSP meeting		
• Other providers and supports/services to be on the IFSP document (e.g., medical home, child care)		
• Time and place preference for IFSP meeting		
• Comfort level with the IFSP meeting and document		

(cont.)

The service coordinator will . . .	✓/✗	Notes
Collaborate to . . .		
• Identify IFSP meeting participants, including providers involved in the child's evaluation		
• Establish meeting time, place, and agenda with the family		
• Facilitate IFSP meeting		
• Enable the family to speak first and often throughout the meeting		
• Enable the family to negotiate for outcomes		
• Develop plan for how families will access supports and resources to meet outcomes		
Perform administrative tasks such as . . .		
• Providing written notice to all involved in the IFSP meeting		
• Acting as the facilitator of the IFSP meeting		
• Ensuring that all forms are correctly completed, signed by, and distributed to all relevant parties		
• Making a copy of the IFSP for a child's file, family, and providers and distribute accordingly (e.g. primary care providers)		

Assisting Families in Identifying Available Service Providers

The service coordinator will . . .	✓/✗	Notes
Share information about . . .		
• The primary provider model		
• The role and competencies of different professional disciplines		
• Strategies for assessing the competence/effectiveness of a service provider		
• The process for identifying members of professional disciplines as service providers		
• Ways to integrate service providers into family and community activity settings		
• Collaborative consultation and transdisciplinary teaming to integrate child's developmental needs across domains, disciplines, and daily learning opportunities and routines		
• Community service providers outside of the EI system		
Gather information from the family about . . .		
• Their knowledge about different disciplines		
• Their preferred time and place for intervention visits		
• Their comfort level with number and frequency of providers		
• Their comfort level with participating in intervention		
• Their comfort level with providing feedback to the interventionist		

(cont.)

The service coordinator will . . .	✓/✗	Notes
Collaborate to . . .		
• Identify a primary service provider		
• Facilitate the choosing of competent service providers for child and family		
• Identify the service delivery structure: time, place, and length of intervention sessions with the family and service provider		
• Identify team meeting times and communication strategies with family and/or service providers		
• Identify how to integrate family's cultural traditions and informal supports within EI		
• Facilitate the sharing of all relevant information (e.g., evaluations, IFSP) across service providers and the family		
Perform administrative tasks such as . . .		
• Gathering necessary documentation on potential service providers		
• Contacting potential service providers		
• Scheduling intervention visits to meet the IFSP outcomes		

Coordinating and Monitoring the Delivery of Available Services

The service coordinator will . . .	✓/✗	Notes
Share information about . . .		
• Agency and provider responsibilities		
• Team process and integration of learning across domains		
• Effective communication strategies across service delivery teams and agency activities		
• How providers should facilitate the behavior and development of the child		
• Criteria by which to measure individual child and family IFSP outcomes progress		
• A system for tracking the delivery of services and intervention sessions		
• Strategies for requesting changes in IFSP and/or service delivery plan		
Gather information from the family about . . .		
• Their satisfaction with the IFSP and service delivery		
• Their confidence in being able to facilitate their child's development as a result of intervention		
• Where and when intervention sessions have occurred		
Collaborate to . . .		
• Establish and coordinate collaborative consultation and team meetings (e.g., via e-mail, phone, or in person)		
• Monitor (or facilitate) the service delivery schedule		
• Monitor data collection from all members of the service delivery team		
• Follow interagency agreements, attend interagency meeting		

(cont.)

The service coordinator will . . .	✓/✗	Notes
• Establish schedule for the sharing of information and/or formal reports on all child and family outcomes		
• Establish a system for the family to provide feedback on the EI service delivery model, the providers, and child and family progress		
Perform administrative tasks such as . . .		
• Establishing data collection strategies on child and family outcomes for all service providers		
• Keeping record of progress from all providers toward IFSP goals		
• Coordinating the 6-month review of the IFSP		

Informing Families of the Availability
of Advocacy Services

The service coordinator will . . .	✓/✗	Notes
Share information about . . .		
• The definition and uses of advocacy		
• Parent resources for advocacy/support (e.g., parent training and information, parent to parent)		
• The use of mediation and due process		
Gather information from the family about . . .		
• Family involvement with resources such as PTI and parent to parent, and other support		
• Family knowledge about their rights, advocacy resources, and due process		
Collaborate to . . .		
• Assist the family to access and use advocacy supports they need		
• Assist the family to use conflict resolution techniques as needed		
Perform administrative tasks such as . . .		
• Assist the team of service providers to use conflict resolution techniques as needed		
• Assist the family to file for mediation/due process if they are dissatisfied with the EI process		

Coordinating with Medical and Health Providers

The service coordinator will . . .	✓/✗	Notes
Share information about . . .		
• Confidentiality and sharing of relevant information, both verbal and written		
• The concept of a medical home, where care is accessible, continuous, comprehensive, family centered, coordinated, compassionate, and culturally effective		
• A child's nutritional needs for growth and development		
• A child's mental health needs		
• Environmental hazards for children		
Gather information from the family about . . .		
• The medical care providers/medical home		
• The child's physical health needs		
• The child's nutritional needs		
• The child's mental health needs		
• The family's medical insurance/Medicaid coverage		
Collaborate to . . .		
• Facilitate the appropriate sharing of medical information/EI information between the child's service providers (EI as well as health care)		
• Educate service providers about the child's medical needs		
• Identify and obtain additional medical/health services that may be needed for the child		

(cont.)

The service coordinator will . . .	✓/✗	Notes
Perform administrative tasks such as . . .		
• Obtain written consent from family to receive and share development, health, and medical records		
• Request child's health and medical records from the appropriate sources		
• Provide health and medical providers with early intervention evaluations and progress notes		
• Establish an ongoing medical/health record system for the child		

Facilitating the Development of a Transition Plan to Preschool Services

The service coordinator will . . .	✓/✗	Notes
Share information about . . .		
• Transition requirements of early intervention		
• Community and specialized services for which child and family may be eligible		
• IDEA preschool (Part B) policies, if appropriate		
• The child's opportunities to participate in community early childhood programs		
• The transition conference to be held at least 90 days prior to transition out of early intervention		
Gather information from the family about . . .		
• Their knowledge of their child's developmental needs, including disability		
• Their knowledge of early childhood community resources for their child		
• Their knowledge of preschool special education, if appropriate		
• Their preference for the child's preschool placement		
Collaborate to . . .		
• Arrange visits of the family to community and/or school placement options		
• Establish members of transition team		
• Schedule transition team meetings at time and place preferred by parent		
• Facilitate transition team meetings		
• Develop a transition plan		

(cont.)

From *Working with Families of Young Children with Special Needs* edited by R. A. McWilliam. Copyright 2010 by The Guilford Press. Permission to photocopy this appendix is granted to purchasers of this book for personal use only (see copyright page for details).

The service coordinator will . . .	✓/✗	Notes
Perform administrative tasks such as . . .		
• Obtaining written consent from family to share information with potential service providers, including evaluation and assessment information and copies of IFSPs		
• Arranging a transition meeting at a time and location convenient for the family; forward current child information to future service providers prior to the transition meeting		
• Notifying local education agency 9–12 months prior to child turning 3 years		

CHAPTER 5

Talking to Families

P. J. McWilliam

Whereas the other chapters of this book discuss strategies for working with families in specific contexts (e.g., during IFSP or IEP development), this chapter addresses the most fundamental aspect of this work—what we say to families at any point in the process. For more than 20 years, even before the passage of early intervention legislation in 1986 (Public Law 99-457), a family-centered approach has been recommended for working with very young children with disabilities and their families (McGonigel, Kaufman, & Johnson, 1991; Sandall, McLean, & Smith, 2000). A major tenet of this approach is the formation of effective family–professional partnerships, wherein a climate of mutual trust and respect leads to shared decision making and interventions specifically designed to address family-identified priorities. Full implementation of this ideal, however, has proven to be far more difficult than first thought (Bruder, 2000).

Although structural barriers (e.g., policies, staff turnover, hours of operation, caseloads) can contribute to difficulties in developing effective family–professional partnerships (Park & Turnbull, 2003), there is growing consensus that interpersonal variables may pose an even greater challenge (Blue-Banning, Summers, Frankland, Nelson, & Beegle, 2004; Dinnebeil, Hale, & Rule, 1996, 1999; McWilliam, Tocci, & Harbin, 1998; Park & Turnbull, 2003). These interpersonal factors have to do with the quality and content of communicative exchanges between families and service providers—what is said, what is not said, and how and when such messages are exchanged. It's about talking with families in ways that promote trust, respect, and a sense of equality.

What's so difficult about talking with families? Janice Fialka, the parent of a child with disabilities, likens the formation of parent–professional relationships to a dance. At the outset, the professional may be eager to hit the dance floor, while the parent may be hesitant to join in the dance at all.

> Here you are, the professional, eagerly awaiting your new dance partner. Your arms are stretched out inviting us, parents, to enter your world. . . . We, as parents, having not chosen this dance, are usually not as eager to join you. We may approach you not with open arms but with tightly folded ones clutched to our chest. . . . We may feel reluctant, ambivalent, and often unwilling. For one thing, if we choose to join you, we have to acknowledge that our child has special needs. We have to acknowledge that we are entering your world—one that is initially unfamiliar and frightening. Entering into our partnership with you demands that we let go of our dreams and begin to build new ones. (Fialka, 2001, p. 22)

Continuing with her dance analogy, Fialka explains that, even after the parent joins the dance, each partner hears different music at the outset. Thus, partners may proceed with a different pace or timing. There may be hesitations, awkward movements, and even stepped-on toes before the dance (i.e., relationship) is smooth.

> Priorities for parents and professionals often differ. It is as if we each have on our own set of headphones and are listening to our own music with its own tune, words, and rhythm. There's the mother song, the father song, the speech pathologist song, the neurologist song, and the teacher song. Sometimes the only song we can momentarily agree on is "Hit the road Jack, and don't you come back no more!" (Fialka, 2001, p. 26)

Parents' uncertainties about their roles and competencies are compounded by the fact that early intervention practitioners frequently don't possess the communication skills needed to invite parents to join them in the dance of partnership and to make parents comfortable, not only in actively participating, but also in occasionally leading the dance themselves (Brady, Peters, Gamel-McCormick, & Venuto, 2004; Winton, 2000). This chapter is devoted entirely to communication skills, for it is only through the words we say that we convey to parents our respect, our understanding, and our sincere desire for them to join us on the dance floor. If we can effectively convey these messages to parents, over time they are more likely to trust us and become more willing, active, and confident participants.

CREATE OPPORTUNITIES FOR INFORMAL EXCHANGE

Much has been written about communication strategies with families during times of crisis, when parent–professional conflicts arise, in preparing for and conducting child assessments, and in developing the individualized family service plan (IFSP) or individualized education program (IEP). What we say to parents and how we say it is, no doubt, important during these specific situations or phases of service delivery. Even so, such times constitute a relatively small proportion of the communicative exchanges we have with families—or at least they should. Among the factors contributing to quality parent–professional relationships identified in the work of Blue-Banning and her colleagues (2004) was the *frequency* of communication. Both parents and professionals participating in their focus groups said that frequent opportunities to talk and exchange information with one another were critical to the development of trusting parent–professional relationships.

The first task at hand, then, in ensuring effective communication with families is to create opportunities for frequent and ongoing conversations. This does not mean scheduling more team meetings, nor does it mean making specific appointments to talk one-on-one with parents to discuss specific issues or make decisions. What is needed are opportunities for more unstructured, informal conversation—not unlike the daily chats we have with colleagues or friends. Although any one such conversation may seem relatively pointless or insignificant, the accumulation of such brief interactions over time serves to strengthen the relationship. So first, we must believe that the time taken away from other activities to engage in informal exchanges with parents is time well spent. And second, we must adjust our work to create such opportunities.

Practitioners who conduct home visits are probably in the best position to create opportunities for informal conversation. This can be done at the beginning of the visit, before on-task conversations get under way, or a few minutes can be reserved at the conclusion of the visit, as paperwork is rounded up and discussions of "next steps" take place. It is important to remember, however, that establishing informal conversations as a regular part of the home visit is the responsibility of the interventionist. Without a specific invitation to engage in such chit-chat, families may operate under the erroneous assumption that the sole role of the practitioner is to work with the child. Family members might try not to interfere, by staying out of the way, limiting what they say to issues directly related to the child's development, or limiting their contributions altogether. If, however, informal exchanges are initiated by the practitioner, parents are given the "go ahead" to talk, and the practitioner's responsiveness to what they say will keep the flow of the conversation going.

Creating opportunities for informal conversations and establishing these exchanges as the norm may be a bit trickier in classroom-based or clinic-based services. Nevertheless, it can be accomplished. In the case of classroom programs, schedules can be adjusted to ensure the greatest flexibility during arrival and departure times. Having sufficient staffing available to free up the teacher for informal conversations with parents is obviously one consideration. Another consideration is to have several centers (water table, big blocks, and pretend play) established and ready for children when they first arrive. Parents may be invited to join their children in one of the activities for a few minutes before leaving, and teachers may circulate from one center to the next, engaging in informal conversation with parents, while supervising and interacting with the children. Making parents feel welcome to join in the activities and to chat is the key here. Many parents may be rushed themselves at the beginning of the day, but may be a little less hurried at the end of the day, so providing additional times for conversation during pick-up time may be important. In nice weather, scheduling outdoor play at the end of the day may be helpful in creating additional opportunities for brief conversations with parents on the playground. Many a meaningful conversation has also taken place in a parking lot, when a teacher or therapist walked a parent and child out to their car. Again, practitioners may need to take the initiative by starting the conversations and, thus, inviting parents to join in.

Home–school notebooks, notes sent in diaper bags, e-mail, and occasional evening phone calls at convenient times for the family are all possibilities for increasing the frequency of communication with families in classroom programs, but these tend to be limited to matters concerning the child. Although useful, these traditional methods of home–school communication (i.e., home–school notebooks) tend to be used more for the purpose of teachers giving information to families than vice versa. If we want to encourage more active parent participation and the type of information sharing described in the remainder of this chapter, face-to-face communication will be far more effective (Hart, Drotar, Gori, & Lewin, 2006).

Clinic-based services provide additional challenges, because visits typically occur no more than once a week, they are relatively short, and therapy sessions are often scheduled back to back, providing little flexibility. If home visits are conducted like clinic visits, these challenges are all found in home visits, too. Under such pressures, it is even more important that clinicians recognize the importance of informal exchanges in the development of productive relationships, as there will be at least some hands-on time with the child sacrificed in creating opportunities for informal conversations with the parent(s). Conversations with parents initiated at the beginning or the close of a clinic visit, however brief, can be quite meaningful and when done routinely as part of each visit, can result in considerable information about the family as a whole and, over time, lead to a more effective parent–professional relationship. I have also witnessed effective inclusion of parents during the therapy session itself, wherein brief conversations with the parent are interwoven with hands-on work with the child. In fact, this consultative approach is most likely to lead to interventions the family can carry out between clinic sessions.

ACKNOWLEDGE CHILD AND FAMILY STRENGTHS

When working with parents, it is easy to slip into the habit of focusing on problems. As human service professionals, we assume that families have come to us for our help. We, therefore, often begin our work by ferreting out areas of need by asking parents questions such as "What are your biggest concerns about your child?"; "What would you like to work on with your child?"; and "How can I be of most help to you right now?" In focusing exclusively on problems, however, we run the risk of implying that parents lack competence without our help and that they could always do better than they are already doing. We may further imply that children are found similarly—and continuously—deficient.

It is difficult, if not impossible, to establish a true partnership if parents perceive themselves to be in a one-down position or, even worse, when they feel that the professional doesn't recognize the strengths that they bring to the table. Especially during the early years, when parents are first adjusting to their child's special needs and learning the ropes of the service maze, the confidence and self-esteem of many parents may be shaken. Recognizing and acknowledging family and child strengths can do much to communicate respect and to convey recognition of equality in the family–professional partnership.

Through surveys, interviews, and anecdotal reports, parents have repeatedly told us that one of the most important qualities that a professional can have is that he or she demonstrates sincere caring about their child (Blue-Banning et al., 2004). Examples provided by parents typically include examples of how professionals recognize their child's abilities, believe in their child's potential, and are dedicated to the child's future development; in short, that they value their child. Of course we will work on helping parents to facilitate their child's next steps in development or assist them in figuring out ways to manage difficult behaviors but, along the way, it is also important to acknowledge explicitly their children's accomplishments (no matter how small) and their positive attributes. In some cases we may be the only ones who, like the parents, can look beyond what the child *can't* do and fully appreciate what the child *can* do.

Compliments about the child should be a part of our everyday interactions with parents and not reserved for formal assessments, IFSP or IEP meetings, or the biannual summary of the child's progress. They should also transcend specific developmental skills to include more general child characteristics. Providing we are good observers, it should be easy to recognize the child's strengths and issue compliments routinely. They needn't be lengthy, but they must be highly individualized to the child and, above all, they must be sincere. Examples might include

"He's just chock full of energy, isn't he?"
"What a happy baby she is!"
"She may not quite be getting it, but just look at how she's concentrating!"
"He's so much fun to be with!"
"He's trying *so* hard."
"Those big brown eyes are just drinking it all in, aren't they?"
"I think I'm falling in love!"

I remember a little boy and his family with whom I once worked. At 18 months of age, Luke had a strangulation accident that resulted in severe anoxia and subsequent pervasive brain damage. He was left with little, if any, voluntary movement or cognitive functioning. One day, after greeting Luke and his mother at the outset of a visit, his mother said something I'll never forget: "You're the only one who talks *to* Luke" she told me. "Everyone else talks *about* Luke to me." It was natural for me to tousle Luke's hair and say hello to him or ask him how he was doing. But it wasn't until his mother said this that I realized the importance of my actions. She taught me an important lesson that day. Since then, I have come to better understand what parents mean when they say how much they appreciate service providers who see their child as an individual or a real person and not just another "case."

I have also experienced the importance of recognizing child strengths from the vantage point of a parent. When our own daughter was an infant, and her delays were becoming increasingly obvious, I discovered one day in her diaper bag a small paper cutout in the shape of an apple. On it was the date and a short note: "Today she noticed her hands!" That little paper cutout meant so much to me. Amid the worries and fears that I was so intently focused on at the time, her child care provider had noticed something worth celebrating. Having someone with whom to share hopes and to celebrate successes can be as important to a parent as having a shoulder to cry on in times of crisis. So, be sure to remember the importance of shared celebration, whether it be a note in a diaper bag, a good news e-mail, or the quick sharing of a funny story about the child's antics in the classroom.

Just as we compliment children, so should we routinely compliment their parents. Again, such compliments need not be big productions of recognition. Less obvious, well-timed compliments can seem more sincere and are often less awkwardly accepted. The important message to be conveyed is that you recognize the parent's contributions to the child's growth, development, and general well-being. Compliments may be related to the parents' resources for supporting their child's development or the specific skills they demonstrate in caring for, interacting with, or teaching the child. They may also include more personal characteristics of the parent that contribute to the overall day-to-day functioning and well-being of the entire family. Here are just a few examples of the types of statements that might be employed:

"Just look at how he's responding to your voice!"
"You're so patient with her. She clearly thrives on it."
"He *loves* this book. What a great find! Where did you get it?"
"You must be doing something right—he hasn't been sick for weeks!"
"Those blocks are just the right size for his hands to grasp."
"You're so good at figuring out what she wants."
"I don't know how you do it—trying to balance so many things at one time."

SOLICIT PARENTS' OPINIONS AND IDEAS

As early intervention professionals, we feel that we are expected to have solutions to matters concerning a child's behavior or development that fall within our domain of professional expertise. We feel that parents rely upon our years of accumulated education and experience to provide sound advice about meeting their children's needs. After all, why would they seek out our services if they did not want the benefit of our expertise?

So, when a parent presents us with a concern about his or her child, we quickly reach into our bag of tricks and offer a tried-and-true solution. If a parent is concerned about the child's not crawling, we may recommend tummy time, wedges, or toys placed out of reach. For aggression, tantrums, or bedtime difficulties, we suggest appropriate methods from our arsenal of behavior management techniques. And for concerns about a child's not talking, we may recommend any number of solutions from sabotage strategies, to sign language, Picture Exchange Communication System (PECS; Frost & Bondy, 2002), or even sophisticated electronic augmentative and alternative communication (AAC) equipment. The words accompanying our suggestions or recommendations will vary, but often include statements such as "What Tokesha needs is [solution]"; "One way of addressing this issue is to [solution]"; "The first thing we need to do here is [solution]"; or "The best approach is to [solution]." Our recommendations may or may not be followed by an attempt to obtain parental agreement to the proposed solution: "How does that sound to you?" or "Is this something you'd like to try?" More often than not, parents will agree to our recommendation, and we will go away feeling as though we have a mutually agreed-upon plan of action.

All too often, however, we realize over time that the agreed-upon plan has not been put into place. Parents may not show up for or cancel therapy appointments, or they may not get around to contacting a recommended resource. Multiple reasons may be offered for not following through with the use of sign language or implementing toilet training, and expensive equipment such as wheelchairs and electronic AAC devices may be abandoned and left to collect dust in closets or garages. Parents' failures to "follow through" with interventions that they agreed upon can be extremely frustrating for professionals, and they may, unwittingly or not, apply further pressure on the parent to follow through. This pressure may, in turn, result in parental guilt or resentment of such pressure being imposed upon them. Either way, the situation can spiral into a less than amicable relationship.

The lack of parental "follow through" in such situations is often because the solution the professional offered wasn't acceptable to the parents in the first place. Perhaps the solution wasn't consistent with their values or beliefs, or perhaps they really liked the solution but didn't have the time, energy, or resources to implement it. If the only decision parents are offered is to accept or reject the professional's recommendation, parents may feel that rejecting it will make them look like bad parents, so they acquiesce.

In a true partnership, we need to encourage more active participation from parents in the formulation of possible solutions. One strategy for doing this is to postpone jumping in with solutions ourselves until after we have asked parents for their ideas. Some simple ways of doing this are to first convey a partnership approach by saying something like, "It sounds as though this is something you'd like to see changed." [Or "Because you have chosen this as an outcome. . . . "] "Let's see if we can put our heads together and figure something out." Then you can ask, "What have you been doing?" and "How has that been working for you?" If this doesn't generate ideas, you may want to take a slightly different tact by asking, "What do you think it would take to [get Sophie to eat on her own; reduce the stress around dinner time]?" Other variations or follow-up questions might include "What has worked for you in similar situations in the past?" or "What do you think it would take to make a difference?" This doesn't mean that we shouldn't offer our own ideas or recommendations but only that we need to solicit parents' ideas first. By listening carefully to their ideas, we can learn much about their values, beliefs, and resources. Such understanding may serve to modify our own suggestions. Even when parents opt for professional-generated solutions, we should make certain to ask sincere follow-up questions such as "How do you think this will fit into your already busy schedule?"; "Do you see any potential difficulties in implementing this idea?; or "In what ways might we need to modify this solution to make sure it works for you, your child, and the rest of your family?"

SEEK UNDERSTANDING

Although we may never truly understand another person's point of view, we can demonstrate a *desire* to understand where they are coming from—what's important to them and why. When working with parents, our efforts to understand their perspectives and to view the world through their eyes is important in demonstrating respect and, over time, achieving trust. After all, how can we say we respect someone if we have not first demonstrated a sincere desire to understand them?

When we ask parents what their concerns are or what their priorities are for their child and family, we are only scratching the surface of understanding. Family concerns and priorities are the end point—the final outcome or manifestation of personal values and beliefs that are, in turn, a product of unique life experiences and the larger culture in which the family is embedded. Again, we can never come to fully understand the origins of parents' motivations, nor would we necessarily want to. Nevertheless, expressing an interest in achieving a more complete understanding of their perspective can go a long way in conveying our respect. A more complete understanding can also help us to provide more effective services (Turnbull, Poston, Minnes, & Summers, 2007).

Let us consider an example of a typical parent priority for a very young child, such as independent toy play. If we take such a priority at face value and provide interventions aimed at independent toy play (e.g., adapted toys or switch-activated toys), we may be successful and meet parental expectations. Parent motivations behind such a seemingly straightforward goal, however, may vary considerably. It may be that their true priority is increased peer or sibling interactions, the ability to get dinner fixed or a load of clothes washed without the child demanding attention, or perhaps that the grandparents would be more accepting of the child if he or she demonstrated such competence. Thus, working on independent toy play may result in missed opportunities for offering additional or alternative interventions that may more readily address their underlying concern. In some instances, our interventions (e.g., parent spends time teaching child to use adapted toys) may actually interfere with the more pressing priority (e.g., time available to prepare meals or wash clothes).

In this example, it may only take a few minutes and a few well-worded questions to ensure an adequate understanding of the parent's underlying concerns or motivations. First, we must demonstrate that we accept the parent's decision to work on independent toy play (e.g., "That certainly sounds like something we could work toward."). Then, we can check for deeper understanding by finding out *why* this is important to the parent. Asking the parent "Why is that important to you?" seems like the most logical question to ask, but asking "Why?" may be perceived as challenging and, thereby, set up defensiveness on the parent's part. A less straightforward approach is usually a safer bet. For example, your follow-up question may be something like "In what ways might it change things for [child's name] or for the rest of your family, if we succeed in teaching him to play with toys by himself?" Along these same lines, asking more specifics about the expected outcome can sometimes deepen understanding. For example, you might ask, "Can you provide me with a picture of what it might look like if we were successful? What specifically can you envision [child's name] being able to do?"

One of the barriers to understanding is infrequent or inadequate communication. In instances like the one described above, it may only require a few extra minutes to achieve a more complete understanding of the family perspective. In other instances, however, significantly more time may be required, whether this be a single, more intense, and longer conversation (e.g., a Routines-Based Interview; see R. A. McWilliam, Chapter 2, this volume) or gathering bits of information here and there through multiple conversations with parents over a period of weeks or months. The important thing is to create opportunities for talking with parents and to ask questions or make statements that convey our desire to see their child and their family through their eyes.

Creating opportunities for understanding means communicating to the parents that you want to know what they are thinking, what is important to them, and that you value their input. This means taking the time out to *listen*. Body language is meaningful in conveying a person's desire to listen and understand, so the early interventionist should be sure to look relaxed and convey that he or she has the time to listen. The professional may, however, need to take responsibility for starting the conversation. It can begin with something that has recently taken place, something that was observed, or something the parent has mentioned on a previous occasion—for example, "You mentioned on Friday that you were going to visit Jamie's grandparents over the weekend. I was wondering how that went." The early interventionist can then listen and, picking up on what the parent says in response, encourage him or her to talk further about issues or feelings conveyed. The temptation to jump in immediately with solutions to any problems raised should be resisted. Listening and understanding come first.

A similar approach can be used to understand the parent's perspective in the case of real or suspected conflict situations with professionals—for example, "That meeting on Thursday felt a little overwhelming to me, with so many people talking about so many different things. I thought you sounded a little concerned, however, when the speech–language pathologist was talking about using sign language with Justin. You didn't say much at the time, but I wanted to check in with you about that. I'm curious to know what you think about using signs with Justin." You'll notice that both this example and the one in the previous paragraph involve an open-ended or implied question. They invite parents to talk about an issue or concern they may have but, especially in the case of using signs with Justin, do not trap the parent into providing a yes/no answer. The parent is provided with the opportunity to say as little or as much as he or she wants to. Along these same lines, the practitioner hasn't made any assumptions about how the parent feels or hasn't stated his or her own opinion first (e.g., that the trip to the grandparents must have been wonderful or that signing with Justin is a good idea).

If parents are responsive to the professional's overtures to listen and understand, it's important for the professional to demonstrate interest in what the parents have to say. Sometimes, all that is needed is appropriate body language (leaning forward, eye contact, head nods) or a few well-timed brief continuers such as "Oh, I see"; "Hmmm . . . "; or "Okay" to keep them talking. At other times, more specific invitations to continue talking may be needed. These may include comments such as "Wow, that's interesting. I never thought of it in that way before"; "Can you tell me more?"; or "This seems really important to you and I want to understand it better. Can you explain it a little further or, maybe, give me an example?" Of course, follow-up questions related to the specific topic under discussion may also be employed to achieve greater understanding. The major point to be made here is to demonstrate interest in the parents' perspective and to encourage them to continue talking, rather than filling in the silences yourself, to make them feel better, or to jump in prematurely in an attempt to fix things.

Nowhere is seeking understanding more important than in the case of parent–professional disagreements. When parents identify unrealistic goals, propose inappropriate interventions, fail to "follow through," or outright reject what we perceive to be needed interventions, our first temptation is to convince them about the "right" approach to take. The "right" approach, of course, is what we ourselves think is best for the child. We fool ourselves into believing that, if we could somehow get families to understand the importance of our recommendations, then surely they would see the light and agree. As a result, we might stop listening and start talking even more—trying to justify, explain, and convince. An unfortunate side effect of convincing, however, may be that parents feels judged, that the interventionist doesn't approve of what they want or what they are or are not doing for their child. It is easy to see how this could jeopardize the relationship. So, when disagreements arise, interventionists should resist the urge to convince: Redirect energy toward understanding, rather than attempting to be understood. Although not always the case, once parents feel as though they have been understood and that their opinions are respected, they are usually far more willing to listen to and consider another point of view (see Items 10–13 in Appendix 5.1 at the end of this chapter). And their perspective often makes sense once it's fully understood.

DEMONSTRATE CARING FOR THE WHOLE FAMILY

Parents seek out and accept our services as a direct consequence of having a child with special needs. It should not be surprising, then, that most parents expect the content of our conversations and the focus of our efforts to be specifically related to strategies for facilitating their children's development. This is especially true during the earliest contacts between a family and a new early intervention professional. Although it is true that information about other family characteristics, functions, and support networks will be beneficial in serving the child, we must be careful not to violate too strongly the family's expectation for the content of our conversations. If they expect everything to be about only the child, and we want to talk about the family, we will need to explain.

How do we convey to families that we adhere to a family-centered approach—that we care about the well-being of the *entire* family and not just their child with special needs? Our philosophy may, of course, be presented to families in the written materials provided upon enrollment. It may also be presented verbally during our initial contacts with them. Even so, relationships that communicate a family-centered approach are not achieved by mere pronouncements of philosophy. Rather, such relationships are achieved in a more personal manner and incrementally through personal interactions that demonstrate sincere caring for all members of the family.

I remember vividly an encounter with my own daughter's pediatrician when she was only a year old. She was a chronically ill infant and we were returning to the pediatrician's office for a follow-up visit after a hospitalization for pneumonia and a serious blood infection. In fact, this had been the third or fourth hospitalization over a period of only a few months. I was exhausted—not to mention extremely worried—but I was wearing my "Brave Mom" face as I always did when talking with her doctors. After the checkup and a matter-of-fact discussion of my daughter's medical needs, the pediatrician paused, looked up at me, made direct eye contact, and asked, "And how are you doing?" He was so sincere with his question! My Brave Mom face nearly melted, but I said, "Fine" and quickly changed the topic. This feeble response did not take away the fact that I heard him say that he cared about me and how I was doing. This caring meant the world to me at that moment, which is why I remember the incident so clearly, more than 25 years after it happened.

Demonstrations of caring don't have to begin with problems. Nor should we ever assume that families are having a difficult time coping or that their child's difficulties are having a negative impact on other family members. Sometimes parents just plain don't want to "spill their guts" to someone whom they don't really know or to do so while they're dealing with more concrete problems. And some parents may never want to. But that doesn't mean we shouldn't show parents that we recognize the potential impacts on the family, that we care about them as well as their child, and that we are prepared to attend to the needs of the family as a whole (Turnbull et al., 2007).

One easy, nonthreatening, and quick way to begin showing parents that we are interested in the whole family is to attend to information we have about parents' personal interests and family activities or events. For example, we can pay attention to what parents say they do for work: Did they have a new job interview? Did they get training on operating new equipment? Did they just return from an out-of-town business meeting or attend a professional training conference? Was their work likely to be influenced by the latest weather conditions? Pay attention to their hobbies or what they do for fun: Did you notice the mother knitting in the waiting room? Did they have to change an appointment time because they had relatives visiting? Were they late for an appointment because a sibling had a soccer game? Did you notice the hand-embroidered pillows on the sofa during a home visit, or family photos of a camping trip, or a bowling bag left in the front hall? Or maybe during your last appointment the parent mentioned something about buying a new car, a relative who was in the hospital, or a sleepover that a sibling was going to have over the weekend. With such information in hand, we can pose the following types of questions in an informal fashion at the beginning or end of a visit:

"How did the camping trip go this past weekend? Did you get caught in any of those rain showers?"

"Did you have a pleasant visit with your in-laws? Did you do anything special?"

"I love the color of that yarn. Do you do a lot of knitting? Are you making it for yourself or is it a gift?"

"Okay, who's the bowler around here? Do you play on a league?"

"How'd your interview go on Wednesday? Does it seem like something you'd be interested in? If you were offered the position, would it change your travel time in the morning and afternoon?"

"You mentioned last week that your mom was having knee surgery. How'd
    that go? Have you been able to spend time with her during her recovery?"
"How's the soccer player [sibling] doing this season? Have you had a chance
    to watch the games?"

You might say that these are the same types of questions we would ask of a
colleague at work or of a friend. That's exactly right. And by asking them of parents we are, one hopes, conveying to them that we want to be their friend too. At
the very least, we are communicating that we recognize them as individuals and
as family members whose interests, roles, and responsibilities extend beyond their
child with developmental disabilities. This is not to say that we are attempting to be
bosom buddies with all parents. We are, however, attempting to create a relationship—a working partnership—with them. In some instances, parents' responses
to such questions may result in our asking follow-up questions. But often the initial
question is all we need to show that we are interested in their lives—that we care.

At other times, we might have opportunities to be more directly responsive
to parents' needs. For example, suppose at the beginning of a visit, a parent comments that the child had difficulty sleeping and was up half the night. At the conclusion of our visit or during pick-up at the close of the classroom day, we might
remember this comment and say something like, "I hope you can take it easy this
evening and get some much-needed sleep tonight. I'll be thinking about you." This
isn't offering any specific help, but it does show the parent that you acknowledge
the impact of their child's sleep patterns on them, the parents, and that you care
about their well-being. It's a start. It may also make the parent more comfortable
in bringing up the topic with you again if the sleep problem continues. If so, you
might then offer to brainstorm with them about some potential solutions.

We can also demonstrate our desire to consider the needs of all family members every time we recommend a new service or intervention strategy. Extending
the above example of the child who isn't sleeping through the night, let's suppose
the parent did want to talk about some solutions. So, you talk with the parent
about what's going on and introduce some tried-and-true techniques as possible
solutions. Before finalizing any decision, however, you raise the issue of potential
impacts on other members of the family. In this case, you might say something
like, "Although this bedtime strategy has been effective with other children, I'm
wondering if you think it's a good match for your family right now. Even if it works
in the end, it will probably mean some extended crying bouts during the night. Not
only is that difficult for *any* parent to go through, but it may also mean more lost
sleep for you. It might mean some lost sleep for your husband and your other child,
too. Is this something that you think you really want to take on right now?"

Even in the case of something as seemingly simple as an intervention for independent spoon feeding or cup drinking, it is both wise and respectful to demonstrate consideration of all family members. Even 5 additional minutes required to

implement an intervention, in the midst of an already hectic schedule, can make a big difference. So you might ask about the influence of the additional time on the family's ability to get out of the house in the morning, the time diverted from the attention required of siblings, or the spouse's ability or willingness to take up the slack. In the case of a new service or therapy, the time demands may be even greater. So you might say something like, "Speech therapy might provide Sammy with a little help in communicating his needs, but I'm wondering if you think this is a good time to begin a new therapy. This is tax season and I imagine this means it's a busy time for your husband at work. You also mentioned last week that your older son is playing soccer now. So, do you think this would work out for you? Or is it something we need to consider more carefully?"

When we first get to know a family, if we convey an interest in the whole family's "ecology," explaining why the whole ecology is relevant, they become used to this idea and even come to expect that we are prepared to discuss all members of the family. Two strategies discussed in this book help to kick-start families' expectations: developing ecomaps (see Jung, Chapter 1, this volume) and conducting Routines-Based Interviews (see R. A. McWilliam, Chapter 2, this volume).

ACKNOWLEDGE AND RESPOND TO FEELINGS

A discussion of talking with families wouldn't be complete without mentioning how to handle parents' expressions of feelings and emotion appropriately. Most people acknowledge that strong emotions accompany the birth of a child with disabilities or the point at which suspicions of developmental delay unfurl into reality. Families know this and so, too, do the professionals who serve them. And yet, these strong feelings often become the elephant in the room that everyone knows is there but nobody talks about. Obviously, bringing emotions out in the open is a frightening proposition, both for the bearer of the emotions (the parents) as well as for the professionals who must respond. It presents a level of intimacy far beyond that found in most business partnerships, but family–professional relationships remain incomplete unless this level of intimacy can be attained.

Once again, I turn to Janice Fialka (2001), as she so eloquently describes the parent's perspective on what she refers to as the "forced intimacy" between families and early intervention professionals:

Because we are sitting with you during one of the most painful and confusing times of our life, we feel thrust into an uninvited and awkward closeness with you. We sit before you at one of our most vulnerable times. You enter our hearts. You hear our guilt and shame. You listen to our inadequacies. You are stung by our salty tears. You are witness to our pain. We may welcome the tender support and practical interventions, but the nature of the circumstances forces an immediate intimacy that is awkward. . . . I'm struck by the fact that we parents sometimes cry in front of people whose last names we don't know. . . . We're not sure what you think of us and our strong emotions. (2001, p. 23)

Fialka goes on to say how helpful it would be if professionals were responsive to parents' expressions of emotion:

> You as professionals have the opportunity to allow us our feelings, even to invite us to "fall apart" once in awhile in the presence of someone who understands and cares. Your compassion and nonjudgmental attitude can be a gift that decreases our sense of isolation, softens our stress. . . . (2001, p. 23)

Unfortunately, many early intervention professionals are no more comfortable responding to parents' strong emotions than parents are in expressing them in the first place. And so, professionals often do not avail themselves of opportunities to provide this gift of compassion to parents. Brady et al. (2004) videotaped observations of routine home visits and coded the type and patterns of talk that took place between early intervention service providers and families. Of the 13,145 verbal behaviors and 2,155 sequential patterns of exchanges between parents and professionals coded, the category of professional verbal behavior that occurred least frequently (less than 1%) was "accepts feelings," which was defined as "accepts or clarifies the feelings of family members in a nonthreatening manner, without judgment or evaluation of feelings." In fact, when families did express feelings, professionals in the study tended to offer solutions to "fix" the problem rather than responding to the parents' actual feelings. Brady et al. offer an example: "One mother with tears in her eyes and nervously biting her nails stated, 'Oh God, I really want her to be able to walk, you know? And, it's like she's not even sitting up yet.' The professional responded, 'Let's get her on the sofa and work on sitting'" (p. 155).

Perhaps professionals are reluctant to acknowledge parents' emotions because they don't view it as their responsibility, or perhaps they lack confidence in their ability to say the right thing, or they fear, that they may say the wrong thing and make matters even worse. So they say nothing. The failure to respond to parents' emotions, however, sends its own message—that their feelings are foolish or unimportant to you. One can only imagine the detrimental effects of such messages on the relationship. Parents' feelings are real, sometimes they are strong, and ignoring them will not make them go away. We must acknowledge the elephant in the room. But what do we say?

First, we must resist the urge to make parents feel better by telling them that things aren't as bad as they seem or encouraging them to "look on the bright side." Doing so only sends the message that their feelings are unreasonable. Second, we must resist the urge to jump in with suggestions to fix whatever is bothering them. We must deal with the feelings before dealing with the content of their messages. Solutions come later but, first, we must validate their feelings. And, finally, it is important to remember that just because you acknowledge parents' feelings, doesn't mean you are responsible for resolving the worries, fears, anger, or sadness they may express.

The specific words we choose to acknowledge parents' feelings depends on what they say, because we want to reflect back our acceptance of whatever emotions they communicate. Suppose, for example, a parent tells us, "It's so hard to listen to her crying and not know what she wants. If only she had some way of letting me know what she needs . . . if she's hungry, or sick, or frustrated. It would be so much easier!" Rather than centering in on the lack of communication skills, first acknowledge the parents' expressed or implied feeling. So, you might respond with, "It must be really hard to hear your child crying and not know what's wrong." Or you might say, "I can only imagine how frustrating or worrisome that must be for you every day. It's difficult enough to deal with a crying child when you *do* know what's wrong and can give him or her what he or she wants." Then, leave a space of silence to provide the parent an opportunity to expand upon his or her feelings. If he or she chooses to continue the conversation, you can continue to reflect his or her feelings and, only *after* the feelings are fully acknowledged and explored (without judgment), you can decide together if you need to work toward a solution or consider the possibility of enlisting additional help. Sometimes all parents want is someone who will listen to, accept, and validate their feelings.

CONCLUSION

The principles of family-centered service provision are put into practice through what we attend to and how we attend to it. This chapter has reviewed primarily the latter. Both infant–toddler professionals and preschool professionals need to heed the appeal for talking to families in a family-centered way. Through informal exchange, which might not occur without planning, professionals can acknowledge children's and families' strengths (see the first two sections of Appendix 5.1 at the end of this chapter). In a system that too often focuses on children's "deficits" and that can make families feel incompetent, this acknowledgment is important. Families do not come to us just as recipients of our friendly manner, however; their opinions and ideas are necessary for the touted partnership to work. When things don't go well, the family-centered professional seeks understanding rather than a defensive position. To talk to families in ways that matter to them, professionals need to show they care for the whole family, perhaps primarily the primary caregiver. In showing concern for the adults in the family, such as parents, emotionally supportive professionals acknowledge and respond to feelings even before responding to the topic of a person's concerns. Together, this package of interactive behaviors creates an effective professional working in the early childhood field; without bonding to the adult family members, the early childhood professional is rendered relatively ineffectual.

REFERENCES

Blue-Banning, M., Summers, J. A., Frankland, H. C., Nelson, L. L., & Beegle, G. (2004). Dimensions of family and professional partnerships: Constructive guidelines for collaboration. *Exceptional Children, 70,* 167–184.

Brady, S. J., Peters, D. L., Gamel-McCormick, M., & Venuto, N. (2004). Types and patterns of professional–family talk in home-based early intervention. *Journal of Early Intervention, 26,* 146–159.

Bruder, M. B. (2000). Family-centered early intervention: Clarifying our values for the new millennium. *Topics in Early Childhood Special Education, 20,* 105–115.

Dinnebeil, L. A., Hale, L. M., & Rule, S. (1996). A qualitative analysis of parents' and service coordinators' descriptions of variables that influence collaborative relationships. *Topics in Early Childhood Special Education, 16,* 322–347.

Dinnebeil, L. A., Hale, L. M., & Rule, S. (1999). Early intervention program practices that support collaboration. *Topics in Early Childhood Special Education, 19,* 225–235.

Fialka, J. (2001). The dance of partnership: Why do my feet hurt? *Young Exceptional Children, 4,* 21–27.

Frost, L., & Bondy, A. (2002). *Picture exchange communication system training manual* (2nd ed.). Newark, DE: Pyramid Education Products.

Hart, C. N., Drotar, D., Gori, A., & Lewin, L. (2006). Enhancing parent–provider communication in ambulatory pediatric practice. *Patient Education and Counseling, 63*(1–2), 38–46.

McGonigel, M. J., Kaufman, R. K., & Johnson, B. H. (1991). *Guidelines and recommended practices for the individualized family service plan* (2nd ed.). Chapel Hill, NC: National Early Childhood Technical Assistance Center & Association for the Care of Children's Health.

McWilliam, R. A., Tocci, L., & Harbin, G. L. (1998). Family-centered services: Service providers' discourse and behavior. *Topics in Early Childhood Special Education, 18,* 206–211.

Park, J. & Turnbull, A. P. (2003). Service integration in early intervention: Determining interpersonal and structural factors for success. *Infants and Young Children, 16*(1), 48–58.

Sandall, S., McLean, M. E., & Smith, B. J. (2000). *DEC recommended practices in early intervention/early childhood special education.* Longmont, CO: Sopris West.

Turnbull, A. P., Poston, D. J., Minnes, P., & Summers, J. A. (2007). Providing supports and services that enhance a family's quality of life. In I. Brown & M. Percy (Eds.), *A comprehensive guide to intellectual and developmental disabilities* (pp. 561–571). Baltimore: Brookes.

Turnbull, A. P., Summers, J., Turnbull, R., Brotherson, M. J., Winton, P., Roberts, R., et al. (2007). Family supports and services in early intervention: A bold vision. *Journal of Early Intervention, 29*(3), 187–206.

Winton, P. J. (2000). Early childhood intervention personnel preparation: Backward mapping for future planning. *Topics in Early Childhood Special Education, 20,* 87–94.

Talking to Families Checklist

Interventionist: _____ Date: _____

Observer: _____

Did the interventionist . . .	✓ ✗ ? NA	Notes
Create opportunities for informal exchange		
1. Structure home visit, classroom schedule, or clinic appointment to allow time for informal conversation?		
2. Take into consideration family's schedule and time constraints (e.g., times for informal conversation are convenient for families)?		
3. Initiate conversations with parents?		
4. Use multiple strategies for communication (e.g., e-mail, personal notes, phone calls)?		
5. Communicate with families frequently—at least once a week?		
6. Keep conversations friendly, light, and emphasize the positive?		
Acknowledge child and family strengths		
7. Compliment the child; acknowledge positive attributes and successes?		
8. Recognize and compliment family contributions to child successes (resources, skills, knowledge)?		
9. Recognize and acknowledge parent contributions to overall family functioning?		

(cont.)

✓ = done at a satisfactory level; ✗ = not done; ? = perhaps done or done but perhaps not at a satisfactory level; NA = not appropriate (e.g., ran out of time).

Did the interventionist . . .	✓ ✗ ? NA	Notes
Solicit parents' opinions and ideas		
10. Ask parents about their ideas or solutions *first*—before offering professional recommendations?		
11. Fully discuss family-generated solutions and be open-minded about their feasibility?		
12. When professionally generated solutions are accepted, check out the viability of such solutions within the constraints imposed on the family by other family tasks and priorities?		
13. Keep enthusiasm for professionally generated solutions in check until fully discussed with and accepted by the family?		
Seek understanding		
14. Use open-ended questions to understand parents' underlying concerns and motivations for selected outcomes, actions, or decisions?		
15. Demonstrate interest in and acceptance of parent's perspective by listening and using appropriate body language?		
16. Maintain a nonjudgmental stance?		
Demonstrate caring for the whole family		
17. Show an interest in the activities of all family members (i.e., work, hobbies, special interests or events) through comments or easy-to-answer questions?		
18. Ask about the impacts of changes in family life (e.g., change in employment, birth of sibling, relocation) on all members of the family?		
19. Ask about the impacts of child behavior, health needs, and therapies on other family members (parents, siblings, extended family)?		
20. Sympathize with any difficulties parents or siblings are experiencing and provide information about potential resources—if the family is interested?		

(cont.)

Did the interventionist . . .	✓ ✗ ? NA	Notes
Acknowledge and respond to feelings		
21. Listen to feelings—sympathizing and employing follow-up questions. Use active listening?		
22. Resist the urge to paint a brighter picture, minimize strong emotions, or to "fix" it?		

CHAPTER 6

Working with Families from Diverse Backgrounds

MARCI J. HANSON and ELEANOR W. LYNCH

Like snowflakes, no two people are alike. Even identical twins learn, grow, and develop personalities that make each one unique. In spite of the many characteristics that all people share, each person differs from all others in multiple ways. The same is true of families. All families are diverse, and diversity is one of the most intriguing parts of being human and of working in early intervention.

As early interventionists and other service providers work with families of children with disabilities, they will encounter families who differ on every conceivable dimension. Family values, communication abilities and styles, and belief systems, among other variables, will exert an impact on the professional/family working relationship. The purpose of this chapter is to assist professionals in establishing partnerships with family members that respect the diversity of the backgrounds and perspectives that families bring to this relationship. This issue has been identified as one of the essential and central principles to strengthening early intervention systems (Guralnick, 2008) and supporting families (Turnbull et al., 2007).

WHAT IS DIVERSITY?

At the most superficial level, diversity can be described by physical characteristics such as skin color, eyes, or hair. Differences in languages spoken, ways of living, and religious beliefs are also characteristics that contribute to diversity. A person's perspective often defines diversity, in that people may be described as "diverse" when their physical characteristics, language, beliefs, and behaviors differ from one's own. What is familiar and conventional to one person might be experienced as quite surprising, confusing, or upsetting to others because it differs from their own life experience. In the United States, the word *diversity* is often used as a way of referring to people of color; however, diversity is not just tied to race, culture, or ethnicity. It is multidimensional, and all of its dimensions are important to understanding families and how they function.

An understanding of diversity is particularly important for early interventionists because of the close relationships that they build with families. Working in families' homes and focusing on issues related to child rearing, family interaction, disability, and health care makes the interventionist privy to some of the most personal, value-laden, and intimate details of family life. It is, therefore, not surprising that early interventionists are likely to encounter diversity daily. It is also not surprising that building relationships might be more challenging with some families than with others. Although recognizing and understanding the dimensions of diversity does not ensure effective practice, it is an initial step in building effective relationships.

Dimensions of Diversity

How families are structured and who is considered to be a family member are dimensions of diversity that might be the starting point for learning more about each family. For instance, is the family comprised of a mother, a father, and children, or does the family consist of a large number of individuals who are related as a tribe or a clan? Sociocultural factors too, such as socioeconomic status, education, and family members' feelings of self-efficacy, provide information about family members' experiences and views of the world. In addition, the many components of culture and cultural identity such as primary language, race, ethnicity, religion or spiritual practices, values and beliefs related to child rearing, gender roles, traditions, aspirations, and family organization are additional dimensions that define each family's diversity (Hanson & Lynch, 2004). The discussion that follows provides a brief examination of these dimensions, and readers are encouraged to consider each dimension in relation to their own personal experience and belief system.

Family Structure and Family Members

Families come in all sizes and configurations. Large families that incorporate brothers, sisters, grandparents, aunts, uncles, and cousins are not unusual. Nor are small families that might be made up of a parent and child or a grandparent and child. Some families might include all of those related by blood, marriage, and adoption as well as "nonrelatives" who are cared about and significant to the family. Other families might be made up of children and a same-sex couple. Although families are traditionally defined as (1) lasting longer than other groups, (2) being intergenerational, (3) including both biological and legal types of relationships, and (4) providing links to a larger kinship network (Klein & White, 1996), individuals might define their families even more broadly. For example, some people might consider their family to be a small but close group of friends who share their lives.

Statistics on U.S. families highlight the range of possibilities. Of the over 73.9 million children from birth through age 17 in the United States in 2007, 68% lived with two married parents (ChildStats.gov, 2008c). Twenty-three percent lived with their mother only, and 3% lived with their father only. Four percent lived in a situation with neither parent present. The picture, however, is not as clear as these data appear to suggest. Children living with two parents who have chosen not to marry or who cannot legally marry because they are of the same sex are not included as living with "two married parents." Likewise, the percentage of children living in blended families cannot be determined because a parent might be a biological, step, or adoptive parent.

The actual family composition and membership, however, may not exert as much influence as does the family's ability to fulfill the functions that society expects families to perform. Many authors have written about family functions (Bristor, 1995; Onaga, McKinney, & Pfaff, 2000; Ronneau, 1999; Turnbull, Summers, & Brotherson, 1984). Drawing from these works (particularly Turnbull et al., 1984), Hanson and Lynch (2004) take a broad view of family roles and responsibilities and suggest that society expects families to provide (1) love and affection, (2) daily care and health maintenance, (3) economic support, (4) identity development, (5) socialization and guidance, (6) support for educational and vocational development, and (7) recreation, rest, and recuperation. For each family, interventionists might want to consider how the structure and membership affect the family's ability to fulfill these tasks. For example, one large, extended family might provide a wide range of resources and support that assists the family in fulfilling all of the functions, whereas another family of the same size and similar membership might consume the material and emotional resources needed to help the family fulfill its responsibilities. Family membership might also affect family functioning. For instance, in many families grandparents provide the resources that enable young families to fulfill family functions and thrive. In other families, however, the grandparents themselves might need considerable care and support, making it more difficult for young families to meet the needs of their children. Blended families might unite in ways that support family functions or they might struggle with tensions that make it more difficult to fulfill family functions. Whatever the situation, the early interventionist's role is to work within the family framework and assist family members to find ways to accomplish their goals.

Sociocultural Factors

Sociocultural factors might result in differences that trigger feelings of discomfort or inadequacy in all involved. Differences in socioeconomic status (SES), education, and self-efficacy between early interventionists and families they serve might be especially challenging (Hanson & Lynch, 2004). For example, a graduate-level early interventionist making a comfortable living who has been reinforced to believe that she has control of her life might find it difficult to empathize with a mother who is uneducated, impoverished, and feels powerless to change her life circumstances.

Poverty limits both educational opportunity and social experience. It also affects all aspects of daily life, as families try to exist in an expensive, competitive, and material world. Furthermore, more than one-third of children who belong to immigrant families are in families considered to live in "baseline basic budget poverty" (Hernandez, Denton, & Macartney, 2007). In the United States in 2006, 17% of children from birth to age 18 were living below the poverty threshold, and 20% of children from birth through age 5 lived in poverty (ChildStats.gov, 2008b). In 2007, 57% of America's children were identified as white, non-Hispanic in origin, 21% were Hispanic, 15% were black, 4% were Asian, and 4% were identified as "other" races (ChildStats.gov, 2008a). Poverty is related to family structure and culture. A larger percentage of children in female-headed households than those living in two-parent households are poor, and black and Hispanic children are more likely to be poor than are white children, regardless of family structure. For those who have not lived in poverty, its impact on daily life and aspirations is impossible to imagine.

Differences in educational level between families and service providers are also common. These differences might make communication more difficult and collaborative planning strained. When they find themselves amid a team of highly trained professionals, some family members might not feel that they have the knowledge or understanding to participate as equal partners and might be embarrassed by their lack of education and social experience. This can also work in reverse. Some early interventionists find parents who are highly educated professionals quite intimidating.

Self-efficacy or the feeling that one is a capable, competent person who is in control of life choices might highlight differences between early interventionists and some of the families with whom they work. All areas of education and social service are based upon a strong belief in and commitment to making a positive difference—helping people grow, learn, and change. So it is not surprising that early interventionists are optimistic and confident that positive change will occur. Poverty and limited education reduce opportunities, minimize rewards, and dampen confidence, making self-efficacy more difficult to achieve.

None of these factors dictate the way any individual will perceive him- or herself or react to life situations. There are many stories of poor children who become wealthy adults and of adults with limited education who become phenomenally successful. However, sociocultural factors such as poverty, lack of education, and a sense of powerlessness are not attributes that support the successful fulfillment of family functions.

Cultural Components and Early Intervention

Cultural diversity is made up of many components. One's race, cultural identity, language, beliefs, traditions, life practices, and other attributes might be material or immaterial to each individual and family. What is important for an early interventionist is determining which of these components are significant to each family and its members, learning how they are expressed, and finding ways of interacting and intervening that fit within the family's cultural framework. The paragraphs that follow discuss some of these cultural considerations; but before that discussion, it is important to address the concept of race. Anthropologists have used race for over 200 years to describe people based upon their physical characteristics (Gollnick & Chinn, 2001). However, as our understanding of genetics and the human genome has expanded in recent years, it is clear that race is not biologically meaningful (Olson, 2001; Smith & Sapp, 1996). Despite the scientific evidence that confirms our universal similarities, the longstanding prejudices based on the notion of race continue to fuel stereotypes and create barriers for those who do not share the "privilege" of round eyes and lighter skin (Hanson & Lynch, 2004). As a result, race continues to be *socially* relevant—a sociocultural factor that affects many families' interactions with systems and the world around them. It is not, however, a determiner of behavior or beliefs.

One of the most significant cultural considerations is each person's or family's cultural identity. For instance, does the family or any of its members have a strong identification with a particular cultural ethnic group? The answer in any family might be surprising. Some families who have been in the United States for years, including some who might be descendants of the original people on this continent, might be highly identified with their origins and think of themselves as "American Indians," "Italians," or "Chinese." Conversely, others who have been in this country or on this continent for many years might view themselves as "just American." They might not feel strongly about their roots or the beliefs and traditions of their ancestors. The same is true for those who are newly arrived. Some might work to maintain their culture of origin, while others might try to shed it quickly to make way for a new life in a new world (Hanson, 2004). Like cultural identity in which there is as much difference within groups and across groups, families also differ within their own boundaries. Older family members might be highly identified with their culture of origin, whereas younger family members might be more highly identified with the dominant culture that they are exposed to at school, on television, and through their peers. Being a teenager might be a much more salient identity than being Vietnamese, Mexican, or Anglo European.

Primary language constitutes another component of cultural diversity. According to data collected by the U.S. Census Bureau in 2000, 18% of the U.S. population older than age 5 speaks a language other than English at home (U.S. Census Bureau, 2008). This figure was up by 4% from the 1990 census, when 14% of the over-5 population reported speaking a language other than English at home. Although the vast majority (92%) of those who spoke a language other than English at home also spoke English "very well," according to data collected in 2000, 8% spoke English less than "very well." The most common languages other than English were (1) Spanish, (2) Chinese, (3) French, (4) German, (5) Tagalog, and (6) Vietnamese. The West and South had the largest numbers of people who spoke a language other than English at home, and they also had the largest number of individuals who were English-language learners. When the language that families speak or are most comfortable in differs from the language of service providers and the service system, the barriers to offering family-centered and family-friendly services can be difficult to overcome. Even those who are fluent in English for daily needs and basic conversation might find that the language of the system—be it education, health care, or social services—is a language of its own that requires translation.

Beliefs, behaviors, and life practices related to family, child rearing, spirituality, independence, time, tradition, ownership, gender, and aspirations are central to one's culture and cultural identity (Lynch, 2004). Each of these areas can have a significant impact on the goals that families have for themselves and their children as well as the relationships that they build with interventionists. It is also these areas in which differences between families and interventionists often arise. However, providing culture-specific information is both misguided and misleading. As stated previously, there is as much difference *within* cultures as there is *across* cultures. Another variation might be a strong identification with a set of religious beliefs. For instance, for some families, being Jewish, Catholic, Muslim, Hindu, or Christian provides their primary cultural identification.

To help professionals think about potential cultural differences without stereotyping, cultural continua have been suggested (Lynch, 2004). Each continuum represents a range of beliefs about a universal value such as interdependence versus individuality or harmony versus control. All people have beliefs about the relative importance of being interdependent versus exerting one's individuality or a preference for harmony versus a preference for control. Individuals can indicate their preferred position on each continuum; however, their position might not be static. It might change as a result of time, life circumstances, or altered beliefs. No position is right or wrong. It simply represents a preference that leans toward one end of the continuum or the other. Consider the continuum that places interdependence at one end and individuality at the other. For some families, it is more important that everyone work together and contributes to well-being than it is to have any one person stand out. As a result, they might be more interested in ensuring that all family members have time together rather than spotlighting and continually focusing on the needs of the child with disabilities. An interventionist might want to build on this by developing activities for the target child that foster cooperation and include all family members.

Another continuum addresses beliefs about respect for advanced age, ritual, and tradition as opposed to an emphasis on youth, future, and technology. Families who lean more toward technology and its possibilities might want support in finding the latest communication technology for their child or information on the most recent medical research that could improve their child's health and functioning. Families closer to the other end of the continuum might be more likely to rely on practices that have been handed down over generations to treat their child or on rituals that provide comfort to the family. For these families, advocating for invasive surgery, for example, might not be the best approach. Each of the continua has implications for interventionists and interventions. Matching the intervention to the family's beliefs and practices increases the likelihood of success. For a more complete discussion of the cultural continua and their application, see Lynch (2004).

Associations among Family Characteristics

Although families can be described according to their structure, sociocultural factors, and cultural-background characteristics, these factors when viewed in isolation fail to reveal a given family's identity or complexity adequately. Some immigrant families, for instance, might maintain strong ties and identity with their native cultural background, whereas others might have assimilated to a large degree with their new culture. Still others might pick and choose from among their cultural options. They might, for example, use educational services in their new community for their children but elect to rely on more native, traditional practices for health and healing.

The power and the opportunities afforded to families also influence their experiences and outcomes. There is little dispute that families who have few support ties with others, who live in poverty, whose education level is low, and who speak a language other than English, will be severely limited in their abilities to gain access to services they need and to provide optimal experiences for their children. These factors might come together powerfully to curtail family choices and options. Such negative transactions can be reversed or prevented if service providers recognize the contribution of these factors to family outcomes and if they endeavor to understand family differences and support families through approaches that are responsive and respectful of family variation.

DEVELOPING AND ENHANCING CROSS-CULTURAL COMPETENCE

One of the standards for effective practice in education, health, and human services is the ability to work effectively across cultures, in other words, to work effectively with people whose beliefs, traditions, world views, language, and physical characteristics differ from one's own. Cultural competence has been defined in varying ways. The definition forwarded by Rorie, Paine, and Barger (1996) in relation to women's health care addresses it in systemic as well as individual terms by describing cultural competence as "a set of behaviors, attitudes, and policies that enable a system, agency, and/or individual to function effectively with culturally diverse clients and communities" (p. 93). Barrera and Kramer (1997), focusing on early interventionists, suggested that it is "the ability of service providers to respond optimally to all children, understanding both the richness and the limitations of the sociocultural contexts in which children and families as well as the service providers themselves, might be operating" (p. 217). We have previously defined cross-cultural competence as "the ability to think, feel, and act in ways that acknowledge, respect, and build on ethnic [socio]cultural, and linguistic diversity" (Lynch & Hanson, 1993, p. 50). Although each of these definitions has a somewhat different emphasis, all can be used as the underpinning for creating more culturally competent systems and services. What is lacking from each one, however, is the clear acknowledgment that cultural competence is a process, not an endpoint. It is not a set of skills that can be checked off a list and considered mastered. Rather, it requires lifelong attention.

Although cross-cultural competence is not fully achievable, there are a number of steps that individuals can take to increase and enhance their skills. The first is *self-awareness* (Barrera & Corso, 2003; Harry, 1992; Lynch, 2004). Our own beliefs, biases, and behaviors are so ingrained that we often fail to recognize that they simply represent our own worldview, not the way that all people view the world. Becoming more self-aware begins with an exploration of one's own heritage including such things as place of origin or indigenous status, migration, languages spoken, political leanings, vocations, religious affiliation, socioeconomic status and educational experiences, and so forth. This process allows one to determine the ways values, beliefs, customs, and behaviors have been shaped by cultural roots and provides the information necessary to determine which views are personal rather than universal.

A starting point for increasing self-awareness is to consider one's own values, biases, and behaviors. It is likely that many of those values and biases were instilled in childhood. Identifying one's values is a first step toward increasing self-awareness. For example, if one places high value on punctuality, self-determination, and achievement, it may be more challenging to work with families who miss or are late for appointments, who have difficulty making decisions, and who do not follow through or use the services that are available. Confronting one's biases also plays a role in increasing self-awareness. Most of us have heard comments that suggested that some groups are better and brighter than others, that some are better athletes than others, that some are cleaner than others, or that some are more American than others. All comments that divide people into groups create biases. Sometimes the bias is positive, but more frequently it is not. As a first step in identifying biases that you may have, consider the comments you make about others, the jokes that make you laugh at others' expense, and the thoughts that you would never admit that flash through your mind when you confront difference. Biases that exist are not easily set aside or compartmentalized. They influence one's work.

A final step in increasing self-awareness is to consider one's behavior in relation to people who do not share a similar background, culture, ethnicity, set of values and beliefs, or socioeconomic status. Think about your own approach to diversity. Do you act in ways that enable you to learn more about others' perspectives and points of view, seek them out as friends, colleagues, and mentors or do you tend to maintain a personal and/or professional distance that does not challenge your own perspective? Each individual who we know enriches our own way of being in the world. Limiting contact to the familiar limits our own possibilities as well as those of others. Understanding oneself is the foundation for increasing cultural competence. The journey into one's self is challenging, but the personal and professional wisdom that can be gained is worth the effort. (For a more complete approach to increasing self-awareness, see the exercise "A Cultural Journey" [Lynch, 2004]).

A second step is to *learn more about others' cultural and sociocultural perspectives*. As stated earlier, ascribing specific attitudes, beliefs, and behaviors to specific cultures is both misguided and misleading. Many differences are found within cultures as well as across cultures. What is true for one individual or family might be quite different for another. Also, culture is dynamic. It is not immutable; rather, it is constantly changing. Given these caveats, how can information about other cultures be gained? Lynch (2004) has suggested the following strategies:

> (1) learning through books, the arts, and technology; (2) talking, socializing, and working with individuals from the culture who can act as cultural guides or mediators; (3) participating in the daily life of another culture; and (4) learning the language of the other culture. (p. 48)

None of these strategies is sufficient, but each can add to the appreciation and understanding of cultural and sociocultural differences.

The third step is to *apply one's self-awareness and the information learned about other cultures in practice*. Taking the risk to explore the family's cultural and sociocultural identities, learning more about their life practices and beliefs, and crafting interventions that support their worldviews can help bridge cultural divides. Applying knowledge to practice takes practice. Through suspending judgments and learning about and accepting the beliefs and practices of others, the interventionists will also refine their own knowledge, skill, and competence.

BUILDING RELATIONSHIPS WITH FAMILIES: RECOGNIZING AND RESPECTING DIVERSITY

Each service provider will have the opportunity to work with a wide range of families. This opportunity and privilege brings with it the responsibility to anticipate and respect the many different styles of interacting as well as values and life practices that families might manifest. Several important dimensions along which families might vary are considered below: styles of communication, beliefs about family roles, views about children and child rearing, beliefs regarding disability or risk conditions, and views about change and interventions (also discussed in Hanson, Lynch, & Wayman, 1990).

Styles of Communication

Successful, culturally responsive, family-centered services require effective communication, which, of course, is essential to the establishment of relationships. Both verbal and nonverbal modes of interaction must be considered. People who have traveled, particularly internationally, can appreciate the challenges of attempting to communicate with individuals who speak a language different from their own. Often, a direct translation of a word or phrase fails to provide understanding or it even might produce a startling event such as an unidentifiable food on one's plate at a restaurant! Challenges might extend to nonverbal forms of communication as well. For example, a gesture in one country, such as an extended hand with fingers motioning toward the greeter or a pat on a child's head, might indicate an acknowledgment or bid for interaction. These same gestures might be seen as obscene or highly inappropriate in another country or context. To the traveler these miscommunications are often the source of humorous experiences. Communication and cultural misunderstandings, on the other hand, might result in a serious breach of confidence between a service provider and family because issues of disability, caring for children, and treatments are so deeply personal and important to families.

Concerns about communication extend far beyond the notion of whether two people speak the same language. The meanings associated with an interaction and the communication styles preferred by individuals influence how well they communicate with one another. Cultures are often characterized along a continuum referred to as high context to low context. In high-context cultures, situational cues are of great importance, and individuals often rely on established hierarchies and prefer nonconfrontational responses. In low-context cultures, communications are typically direct and to the point, with an emphasis on use of speech. The dominant Anglo American culture is an example of a low-context culture. In the many more high-context cultures, on the other hand, it is not so much what is said that is important, but how it is communicated. In fact, what is left unsaid might be more important than what is spoken. For the service provider and family alike, this can be confusing or result in misunderstandings. A service provider, for instance, might recommend an intervention. The family member might respond by nodding his or her head up and down. To the service provider, this means that the family member agrees with the recommendation. However, the family member might be merely acknowledging that the message was heard—not necessarily that he or she agreed with or intended to act upon the recommendation.

Issues of who is greeted and how they are greeted also are important to building relationships. Cultures will vary as to whether fathers or mothers or elders or parents should be first addressed to show respectful greetings. Also the manner in which family members are addressed, such as the use of a formal name as opposed to a more casual greeting (first name), can affect the beginning interactions. Likewise where and how one sits or stands, one's appearance and style of dress, and the use (or not) of touch such as a handshake, are all governed by cultural mores. Service providers are well-advised to proceed cautiously initially, gathering as much information about the families' preferences prior to any meeting and following the family's lead in terms of style when the meeting does take place.

For many, if not most, families, it is stressful to be constantly required to interact with a wide range of professionals in order to acquire services for their children. For some, having a child with a disability might be considered shameful in their culture. Thus, the mere act of being identified or interviewed and questioned about the disability or service might bring discomfort. For these family members, the public disclosure of these issues might be considered a disgrace. These families might prefer a more indirect method of gathering information and one that occurs over a longer period rather than in an initial-interview situation. In such circumstances, working with a cultural guide or mediator, such as a bicultural individual who travels in both the native and the new service environment can be essential in establishing common ground and understanding with families.

Families too might differ as to their expectations for the type of information they wish to receive from professionals as well as the methods through which it is delivered. Some families expect answers and direction from professionals, and they might see the professional as incompetent or uninterested if they do not provide these specific recommendations. On the other hand, for other families a more directive approach is offensive. A family-centered approach to working with families has often been interpreted as asking families to identify what types of services they want. Even that interpretation is misguided, but members of the dominant culture who speak English and are familiar with service systems might feel comfortable and confident in identifying services they want or might, in fact, demand to be involved in this fashion. Other families, who might be new to this culture and service system, might find the options baffling at best or offensive and inappropriate to the child and family's service needs. Again, gaining some understanding of the family's background and experiences prior to initiating services will help the service provider begin the interaction on a more culturally respectful footing.

Service providers, thus, are cautioned to become knowledgeable about the family's preferences and cultural styles of communication in order to gather information from them and identify intervention goals and approaches more effectively. In some instances, this information will come from other professionals who have or are working with the families. Early interventionists and service providers also should ask families what they prefer rather than make assumptions based on their own values or on the family's race or language. Often other professionals, who are also members of the cultural group, can serve as cultural mediators or guides to provide tips on effective means of communication. The reader is also referred to chapter summaries in Lynch and Hanson (2004) for specific suggestions on cultural courtesies and customs that will assist service providers in establishing working relationships and effective communications with members of various cultural groups found in the United States. This information is provided on many of the major cultural/ethnic groups in the United States with an extensive discussion of each group.

Beliefs about Family Roles

As previously discussed, families differ in terms of how they define family membership. For some it might mean a parent and a child, whereas for others the family will be a large number of individuals in a tribe or clan who might not always be directly related by bloodlines. The meaning attached to "extended" family members varies considerably. Although differences by region exist, in the dominant culture in the United States, family members other than parents or guardians often play a less significant role in defining goals and services for children. In many other cultures, however, kinship networks are all-important, and large extended networks of individuals in the family share responsibilities for all family functions such as child care and rearing and rely on one another for primary support. The service provider might not begin with much credibility or importance in the eyes of family members. This might be a difficult role to assume, particularly for interventionists who are accustomed to being regarded as experts in their fields of practice.

Families differ, as well, in the assignment of roles based on gender and status. Whereas mothers often are primary caregivers, particularly for young babies, this might not be the case for all families. Grandparents and older siblings or other relatives might play vital roles or even provide primary caregiving. Differences with respect to decision making regarding child rearing and treatments, too, are found across families. In some cultures the mother will be the primary decision maker, whereas in others it will be the father, elder, grandparent, or tribal or clan chief. The service provider is advised to avoid making a priori assumptions about which family member should or should not participate in decision making. Failure to show respect for the decision maker or to work within the family's definition of roles might result in families' electing not to participate in the service system. Valuable sources of support for any intervention are found in these kinship networks.

Views About Children and Child Rearing

Throughout history and across cultures, the status and role of children has varied considerably and runs the gamut from that of precious treasures or gifts from God, to burdens, to a family's means of support. Today the dominant culture in the United States is quite youth oriented, and children are typically valued and indulged and even accorded great power in the economic marketplace. In this culture individuality is typically fostered, in contrast to many other cultural perspectives in which conformity to cultural standards and norms is most highly valued. Thus, service providers will encounter many differences in families' styles of caregiver–child interaction, caregiving values and standards, and views regarding the role of children.

For many groups the early years are a time of close contact between the mother and child, and the child's dependency needs are immediately met. However, changes in family roles, particularly with the great number of parents in the workforce, have broadened the range of individuals who provide early care to infants. As children grow older, people shift their expectations for children's behavior. Whereas some cultures continue to provide indulgence and gratification to the child for many years, others demand more independence and expect children to assume more responsibility. Thus there is a shift from primarily child-focused interactions and the fostering of dependence in the earliest years to expectations of more independence. Yet the ages at which children are expected to conform to cultural norms might vary. For service providers who are governed by developmental milestone charts that dictate when children "should" be toilet trained or demonstrate independent feeding with a spoon, their abilities to provide culturally sensitive services will be challenged. Failure to respect families' long-standing cultural values about what constitutes "good" and "bad" child behavior, appropriate child developmental norms, and parental or caregiver responsibilities and practices, could jeopardize the service provider's ability to build an effective working relationship with the family. The values and cultural preferences of the family must be paramount in effectively developing a program for the child.

Beliefs Regarding Disability or Risk Conditions

Whereas service providers have received training and acquired knowledge regarding the characteristics and causes of disabilities and risk conditions, their views might be at odds with the perspective of a given family or particular cultural group. Great variation exists in the attribution assigned to these conditions. For many people, the disability or risk condition will be ascribed to a random event, and the family is required to adjust or adapt to the modified expectations and needs of the child. Some families emphasize the role of fate. They might believe that the disorder is the result of bad luck or family misfortune. For others, the condition might be attributed to a transgression of the mother or father or even ancestor or to something a member of the family didn't or did do during a pregnancy, such as something the mother ate. For some, the disorder is explained as the individual's possession by ghosts, demons, or evil spirits.

The family's interpretation of the disability or risk condition is influenced by whether they view themselves as responsible or culpable for the condition. When the responsibility is in some fashion seen as resting with the family, the family might experience great shame or stigma as a result of having a child with a disability or risk condition.

Learning how families interpret disability and information about disability is not always easy. It can, however, be aided by knowing more about their culture in general and their values, beliefs, and biases as a family. An early intervention/service provider can glean this information by actively listening to families. Open-ended questions to family members that ask them to describe their child and their child's circumstances and condition will be useful in developing knowledge and appreciation of their values and beliefs. Working with a cultural mediator can also increase the interventionist's understanding of the family's perspective. Understanding the family's perspective is essential to developing an effective working relationship and to establishing culturally responsive services.

Views about Change and Interventions

Linked to perspectives regarding disability and risk are family views regarding change and intervention. Families who ascribe to fatalistic explanations for the disability or risk condition might believe that no intervention is needed or possible and they might be reluctant to seek services. Likewise, those who attribute causation to a family transgression are likely to avoid services or assistance outside the immediate family because of the shame or stigma associated with the condition. Often service providers are frustrated or upset because these families elect to accept their fate or avoid help-seeking rather than make active attempts to remediate or modify the condition. These views are in sharp contrast to families that understand the disorder as a random event and elect to participate in the wide array of services that are offered in education, health care, and social service systems.

One area in which cultural perspectives are particularly salient is that of health care. Dominant culture views typically show great reverence for new technologies and intervention approaches that "fix" or attempt to remediate the condition, such as surgeries, drugs, and therapies. This view can be at odds with more fatalistic cultures or cultures that take a more holistic approach to the individual and see a direct link between mind and body. For many cultural groups, treatment approaches are aimed at achieving more balance between mind and body or physical and social factors, rather than treating just the physical symptoms. The choice of the interventionist, healer, or service provider, or which one is really listened to, will be influenced by one's perspective. Folk healers or elders might place the family in a much more central role in treatment than do western doctors or other health care personnel. These healers might promote more holistic approaches that involve herbs, massage, and sometimes even the use of plants and animals to treat the underlying condition. Community service providers might experience these treatments as foreign or even bizarre or, in some cases, even harmful. Regardless, an understanding of the meaning families attach to change and treatment is essential. Service providers are well-advised to become more knowledgeable about families' beliefs and practices and to incorporate traditional family methods (e.g., use of amulets, work with folk healers) into mainstream service system interventions as much as possible. A memorable book *The Spirit Catches You and You Fall Down* (Fadiman, 1997) elucidates the importance of this understanding and the potential for cultural mismatches when service providers and families differ in beliefs and fail to communicate or learn about one another adequately.

Appreciating the many different values, beliefs, and practices to which families adhere is central to developing effective working relationships and partnerships. Given the diversity of the country's population, service providers will have the opportunity to meet and work with families from a wide range of backgrounds. Certainly many families will be similar in perspective and style to the service provider, and little adaptation will be required by either party to begin communication and relationship building. In other instances, however, these differences in values and life practices might leave the service provider feeling ineffectual or, in more extreme circumstances, even repulsed or at odds with families. Skilled family-centered service providers build trust with families by respecting differences, taking time to learn about family preferences and priorities, and not passing judgment. The previous discussion has highlighted a few dimensions upon which families might vary. Considering these dimensions and others will assist service providers in getting off on the right foot with families as they begin building a relationship.

PARTNERING WITH FAMILIES TO DEVELOP AND ADDRESS GOALS

Creating More Culturally Competent Systems

Early childhood special education relies on family-centered approaches that require interventionists to build strong, trusting relationships with families. As previously noted, these relationships are foundational to creating family–professional partnerships that enable families and professionals to work collaboratively in all aspects of intervention. However, if the early intervention program or system is not culturally responsive, it is far more challenging to build those relationships. Like cars, systems sometimes need a tune-up or at least a checkup to see if policies, procedures, and practices encourage cultural competence. Appendix 6.1 at the end of the chapter includes some general questions to ask as interventionists, administrators, and representative family members review their programs.

In addition to ensuring the system is functioning in ways that are culturally competent, it is also important to review each component of service delivery. Education, health care, and social services all rely on a predictable process for initiating, delivering, and evaluating services (Lynch & Hanson, 2004). The components typically consist of (1) initial contact and an exchange of basic information; (2) data gathering and assessment; (3) development of an intervention plan; (4) plan implementation; and (5) monitoring and evaluation of child, family, and program outcomes. Each is discussed in the paragraphs that follow in relation to cultural competence.

Initial Contact

Most people approach calling an unknown professional about a concern with trepidation. Consider how much more difficult that must be for individuals who are not fluent in the language of the service system, have limited experience with professional services, have limited resources, or are in the country without proper documentation. Add to that the fact that families are contacting early intervention programs because of serious concerns about a child whom they love dearly. This initial contact is the family's first impression of the program and its services, so it is essential that the experience be positive. The individual who takes the call is the program's "first responder," and, like first responders in fire, police, and emergency medical services, it is critical that he or she be well trained. Unfortunately, this pivotal role is often assigned to someone with no professional training, or far worse, to an answering machine. All first responders in early intervention should be trained, coached, and monitored to ensure that they are listening to families' requests and concerns, responding in supportive and caring ways, and following through without delay to help the family take the next step in the process. If paperwork is required, the first responder should determine in which language it should be provided and offer the support in completing it. This might also be a time when offering to link the family with a trained parent facilitator who shares their language might be a way to provide support, but it cannot be assumed that speaking the same language guarantees that values and worldviews will be shared.

Data Gathering and Assessment

Data gathering and assessment are often rigidly prescribed regardless of their appropriateness for individual children and families. The first consideration is the language in which commercially available tests are written and administered. If it is not the language of the child or family, results cannot be assumed to be accurate or of value in planning the intervention. Although one would assume that no one would administer a test in a language that a child did not understand, direct translations of the test are no better. It is also quite common for children growing up in bilingual homes to know some words such as the words for family members in one language and other words such as colors in another (Barrera & Corso, 2003). As a result it takes a skilled assessor along with information provided by parents or caregivers to determine a child's functioning.

The tasks included and measured in typical assessments might also need to be considered in relation to the child's cultural and sociocultural experience. Turning pages of a board book might not be within all children's experience, and some children might be unable to respond as expected for their age level. Other children might have had little structure in their lives and find it difficult to respond to directions. Still others might have had little experience with individuals outside their family or cultural group and might find it difficult, if not impossible, to respond to a stranger.

Arranging the assessment at a time that allows family members to bring those close to the child, conducting the assessment in the home, using only one assessor, including family members in administering items, and minimizing the length of the session might help the child and family feel comfortable. Many assessment items that have obvious value to interventionists might seem strange to families. Thus, the professional's explaining the purpose of each item being administered and the family's observing each behavior can help build the bridge between family members and early interventionists. Working with an interpreter is, of course, essential if the family's preferred language is not the language of the assessor.

Another way to build the bridge between families and interventionists is to focus assessment initially on those areas about which the family has expressed a concern. If they are worried that their 17-month-old daughter is not able to walk, interventionists should begin with that developmental area rather than another. Learning more about the family and their concerns, priorities, and resources is another part of the data-gathering process. To work with the family as partners, it is important to learn about their concerns, views on child rearing, traditions, and daily practices. Unfortunately, this is not the kind of information that can be gathered before a relationship with the family has been established. It is also not the kind of information that should be gathered using a checklist. Rather, a series of conversations when family members feel comfortable reveals the most comprehensive and helpful information that can be used to tailor interventions to fit family preferences. Table 6.1 lists the kinds of information that can be gathered in informal conversations that will help determine how interventions can be optimally structured.

Developing an Intervention Plan

Early intervention in the United States places a high value on parent–professional partnerships in developing child and family goals and intervention plans. Viewing family members as equal partners is not, however, a common perspective in many other cultures. Both cultural and sociocultural factors, such as putting teachers on pedestals and having a limited education, respectively, might make it difficult for

TABLE 6.1. Guidelines for the Home Visitor

Part I—Family structure and child-rearing practices

Family structure
- Family composition
  - Who are the members of the family system?
  - Who are the key decision makers?
  - Is decision making related to specific situations?
  - Is decision making individual or group oriented?
  - Do family members all live in the same household?
  - What is the relationship of friends to the family system?
  - What is the hierarchy within the family? Is status related to gender or age?

- Primary caregiver(s)
  - Who is the primary caregiver?
  - Who else participates in the caregiving?
  - What is the amount of care given by mother versus others?
  - How much time does the infant spend away from the primary caregiver?
  - Is there conflict between caregivers regarding appropriate practices?
  - What ecological issues impinge upon general caregiving (housing, jobs, etc.)?

Child-rearing practices
- Family feeding practices
  - What are the family feeding practices?
  - What are the mealtime rules?
  - What types of foods are eaten?
  - What are the beliefs regarding breastfeeding and weaning?
  - What are the beliefs regarding bottle feeding?
  - What are the family practices regarding transitioning to solid food?
  - Which family members prepare food?
  - Is food purchased or homemade?
  - Are there any taboos related to food preparation or handling?
  - Which family members feed the child?
  - What is the configuration of the family mealtime?
  - What are the family's views on independent feeding?
  - Is there a discrepancy among family members regarding the beliefs and practices related to feeding an infant or toddler?

- Family sleeping patterns
  - Does the infant sleep in the same room or bed as the parents?
  - At what age is the infant moved away from close proximity to the mother?
  - Is there an established bedtime?
  - What is the family response to an infant when he or she awakes at night?
  - What practices surround daytime napping?

- Family's response to disobedience and aggression
  - What are the parameters of acceptable child behavior?
  - What form does the discipline take?
  - Who metes out the discipline?

- Family's response to a crying infant
  - Temporal qualities—How long before the caregiver picks up a crying infant?
  - How does the caregiver calm an upset infant?

(cont.)

TABLE 6.1. *(cont.)*

Part II—Family perceptions and attitudes

Family perception of child's disability
- Are there cultural or religious factors that would shape family perceptions?
- To what, where, or whom does the family assign responsibility for their child's disability?
- How does the family view the role of fate in their lives?
- How does the family view their role in intervening with their child? Do they feel they can make a difference or do they consider it hopeless?

Family's perception of health and healing
- What is the family's approach to medical needs?
- Do they rely solely on Western medical services?
- Do they rely solely on holistic approaches?
- Do they use a combination of these approaches?
- Who is the primary medical provider or conveyer of medical information? Family members? Elders? Friends? Folk healers? Family doctor? Medical specialists?
- Do all members of the family agree on approaches to medical needs?

Family's perception of help-seeking and intervention
- From whom does the family seek help—family members or outside agencies and individuals?
- When the family seeks help, does it do so directly or indirectly?
- What are the general feelings of the family when seeking assistance—ashamed, angry, demand as a right, view as unnecessary?
- With which community systems does the family interact (educational, medical, social)?
- How are these interactions completed (face-to-face, telephone, letter)?
- Which family member interacts with service systems?
- Does that family member feel comfortable when interacting with service systems?

Part III—Language and communication styles

Language
- To what degree . . .
  - ○ Is the home visitor proficient in the family's customary language?
  - ○ Is the family proficient in English?

- If an interpreter is used,
  - ○ With what culture is the interpreter primarily affiliated?
  - ○ Is the interpreter familiar with the colloquialisms of the family members' country or region of origin?
  - ○ Is the family member comfortable with the interpreter? Would the family member feel more comfortable with an interpreter of the same sex?

- If written materials are used, are they in the family's native language?

Interaction styles
- Does the family communicate with each other in a direct or indirect style?
- Does the family tend to interact in a quiet manner or a loud manner?
- Do family members share feelings when discussing emotional issues?
- Does the family ask you direct questions?
- Does the family value a lengthy social time at each home visit unrelated to the early childhood services program goals?
- Is it important for the family to know about the home visitor's extended family? Is the home visitor comfortable sharing that information?

some families to participate fully in developing the intervention plan. They are not used to, do not expect, and do not prefer to take such an active role. In addition to these factors, many families find it intimidating to be surrounded by well-acquainted, highly trained professionals in the planning meeting. It is not surprising that the greater the cultural or sociocultural differences, the more intimidating it might be.

To make this part of the process more comfortable for families, interventionists should brief them about the meeting before it takes place. If family members know who will be involved and what they will be presenting, the meeting itself might be more comfortable for them. Tailoring the meeting agenda and style to family preferences also will aid in ensuring family comfort and participation. Helping families formulate their own questions, which they or a professional might ask, is another strategy for expanding their role. As with the assessment, limiting the number of professionals present and encouraging families to bring people who are important to them can help reduce anxiety. Allowing time for questions is also important. If a family doesn't have any questions, it might be helpful for professionals to talk about some of the questions that often come up in these meetings. In that way, families might have their questions answered without having to ask.

Planning meetings is seldom easy, as a lot of information is given in a limited time; however, every effort to make families comfortable and professionals unhurried is worthwhile. Gestures that show respect for families such as taking time to get better acquainted before rushing into reports, serving coffee or tea, and ensuring that the person who knows the family best is seated next to them will encourage families to become more active partners.

Implementing the Plan

Plans not implemented cannot succeed, so developing implementation strategies that fit within the family's beliefs, values, and resources is crucial. If families did not agree with the established goals but were too polite to say so, implementation is unlikely. Families' goals might change as circumstances change. Although self-feeding a young child seemed like an important goal a month ago, family members have decided that they do not have the time or that it is too messy now that grandmother is babysitting at her house. Because developmental issues are so often the focus of early intervention, and cultural perspectives on "normal" development and child-rearing practices differ, differences between the interventionist's and family's expectations are possible.

One strategy for improving the fit among family priorities, goals, and outcomes is to ensure that the selected goals (or "outcomes" on individualized family service plans [IFSPs]) are those that are most important to the family. Involving parents, grandparents, brothers, sisters, aunts, uncles, and cousins with parental permission can extend a child's opportunity to practice new skills and behaviors. Adapting goals and outcomes to family and community preferences such as eating with chopsticks instead of a spoon and fork or behaving in cooperative rather than competitive ways can encourage intervention by families and success.

Monitoring and Evaluation

Determining whether a child has met the targeted goals and whether family members are satisfied with the extent to which they have met their outcomes is a significant component of program implementation. Without data on success and satisfaction, it is difficult to make meaningful changes. Data on child outcomes are generally easy to collect. Collecting information from families about their experiences with the program and suggestions for improvements is more difficult. Because most families of young children in early intervention programs provide favorable feedback, it is often difficult to get information that will lead to program improvement. One strategy that can be used to collect more meaningful data is to sponsor roundtables led by other parents or community leaders. Without staff present, the community facilitator can ask family members to describe what they like best and least about the program and what they would like to recommend to programs just getting started.

All aspects of service delivery should be reviewed for their cultural responsiveness. Although these reviews should be ongoing, they are essential every time there is a change in the demographics of the families served and in the composition of the staff. As rules, regulations, and legislation governing service delivery are created, it becomes necessary to consider their impact on culturally competent service delivery. In addition to the suggestions provided in this section, Appendix 6.2 at the end of the chapter provides some questions that administrators, staff members, and families can consider as they examine a program's cultural competence.

Special Considerations in Home-Based Services

Services for infants and toddlers are often provided in families' homes. The intimacy of this form of service delivery cannot be overestimated. In almost no other service do professionals work within the home, with the child as well as the family, and with issues that are as personal and value-laden as child rearing. The level of trust that families place in early interventionists is extraordinary. Professionals, therefore, must adopt the strictest codes of both ethical and respectful behavior. Ethics are principles of appropriate conduct that are part of every profession. In early intervention, they include behaviors such as maintaining confidentiality, working only in areas of one's expertise, and respecting family decisions.

In addition to fulfilling the ethical standards of the profession, respect for each family and its members is required. The trust that families place in interventionists must be reciprocated with respect. Respect can be given in many ways. Everything from removing one's shoes when entering some homes, speaking to the eldest family member first, or accepting family decisions that differ from recommendations is a sign of respect. Given the trust that families place with interventionists, respect is little to ask in return.

ACHIEVING RESPONSIVE AND EFFECTIVE SERVICES FOR FAMILIES FROM DIVERSE BACKGROUNDS

Issues of diversity can seem overwhelming. Service providers might feel hesitant and nervous as they endeavor to establish effective working relationships and partnerships with families whose cultures and styles differ markedly from their own. While missteps will undoubtedly occur, entering the relationship with an open heart and mind and honestly attempting to communicate and understand the family's perspective will go a long way toward building trust. The following vignettes demonstrate the importance of these issues. Consider for a moment the two situations that follow.

Situation 1

Shannon was an early interventionist in a large suburban city. Her job entailed visiting families in their homes to provide family-centered services for young children with disabilities who ranged in age from birth to 3 years. She had been employed in this field for over a decade and felt confident in her abilities. Recently, she had to do some extra personal soul-searching and reflection to work effectively with one particular family. This family recently emigrated from the Middle East. Shortly after arriving in the United States, the mother gave birth to a son with spina bifida, and this boy was assigned to Shannon's caseload. Shannon was frustrated and frankly upset by many aspects of the family's life. She couldn't believe that the mother, Aziza, was hardly allowed to leave the house and, when she did, she was required to be covered. Shannon was amazed that it did not seem to bother Aziza that her husband made all the decisions and that her life was primarily spent cooking, cleaning, and washing up after the other family members. Shannon too was concerned that Aziza spent so little time promoting her son's growth and development at home and that her husband seemed to be gone all the time and relatively uninvolved in the child's care.

Situation 2

Carlos was an early childhood special education teacher who had been teaching for 5 years. He spoke both Spanish and English and often had bicultural and bilingual children in his class. This year a child with Down syndrome was placed in his class. The child never spoke, and Carlos was not sure at the beginning what language the child understood, although Carlos was aware that the family was from Southeast Asia. The child's mother and father appeared to be nice enough people, but they asked no questions and never visited the classroom. In fact it took numerous attempts to schedule the child's individualized education program (IEP) meeting, made even more difficult by the need for an interpreter. The mother and father attended the meeting but said very little. Carlos had difficulty understanding why this family was so uninvolved given that their 4-year-old daughter never spoke and clearly had a disability!

In both of these situations, the service providers felt uncomfortable with the behavior of family members regarding the children with disabilities. Establishing an effective working relationship and a family–professional partnership was a challenge in both cases. However, clashes were avoided because both professionals made the effort to reflect on their concerns and gather more information. Shannon, through discussions with her colleagues, worked through her feelings about the role of women in the family and about the priorities this mother had that were in sharp contrast to most of the other mothers in Shannon's caseload. Carlos learned that his family truly cared about their youngster, but that they were working three jobs—the mother worked the day shift and had another job in the early evening and the father worked a long night shift. They relied on two older daughters to look after the preschooler and tend the house. The family simply didn't have the money or resources to do anything else. Neither family spoke English well and had great difficulty communicating with the service providers. Both teachers worked with interpretation and translation services in their communities to both speak with the parents and provide them written materials. Both teachers also consulted with individuals in their communities who were knowledgeable about families with Middle Eastern and Asian backgrounds, respectively. These individuals served as cultural guides and helped Shannon and Carlos to understand the values and lifestyles of the families with whom they were working.

The families in these vignettes differed from the service providers in terms of their languages spoken and cultural backgrounds. Their views about child rearing, family roles, and intervention were potentially at odds with the expectations of their service providers. In both cases the families also were restricted in terms of their power and opportunity to gain access to services and to participate in the larger community. These families could easily have been lost in the system or offended by some of the typical practices in the dominant community of their new environment.

The service providers in these cases took the time to understand the families they encountered and to learn about the family members' preferences and the ways in which they were comfortable communicating. They also worked with knowledgeable individuals in their communities who were able to serve as guides to the cultures and practices of the families that appeared foreign or uncaring at first glance to the service providers.

FINAL COMMENTS

This chapter has highlighted some crucial areas that providers might consider as they begin to build working relationships with families. These include gathering information about families' concerns and priorities and acknowledging and understanding that families' values and practices might differ, even radically, from those of the dominant or familiar cultural group. Tapping other community resources is also essential. By navigating through service systems with particular expertise such as working with families from particular immigrant groups, the homeless, or the working poor, service providers can extend their knowledge and better serve the families assigned to their care. Perhaps the most important steps are for service providers to achieve clarity about their own values and beliefs and recognize when they feel uncomfortable working with a family whose life style and goals are different. Recognizing that neither party is right or wrong and embracing the opportunity to learn new ways of relating can lead not only to great personal growth but also direct one down the path to providing more culturally responsive and family-centered services. Accepting people for who they are and what they bring in background and experience is essential to this communication process.

REFERENCES

Barrera, I., & Corso, R. M. (with MacPherson, D.) (2003). *Skilled dialogue: Strategies for responding to cultural diversity in early childhood.* Baltimore: Brookes.

Barrera, I., & Kramer, L. (1997). From monologues to skilled dialogues: Teaching the process of crafting culturally competent early childhood environments. In P. J. Winton, J. A. McCollum, & C. Catlett (Eds.), *Reforming personnel preparation in early intervention: Issues, models, and practical strategies* (pp. 217–251). Baltimore: Brookes.

Bristor, M. W. (1995). Individuals and family systems in their environments (2nd ed.). Dubuque, IA: Kendall/Hunt.

ChildStats.gov. (2008a). *America's children in brief : Key national indicators of well-being 2008, demographic background.* Retrieved August 12, 2008, from *www.childstats.gov/pdf/ac2008/ac_08.pdf.*

ChildStats.gov. (2008b). *America's children in brief: Key national indicators of well-being 2008, economic circumstances.* Retrieved August 12, 2008, from *www.childstats.gov/pdf/ac2008/ac_08.pdf.*

ChildStats.gov. (2008c). *America's children in brief: Key national indicators of well-being 2008, family and social environment.* Retrieved August 12, 2008, from *www.childstats.gov/pdf/ac2008/ac_08.pdf.*

Fadiman, A. (1997). *The spirit catches you and you fall down: A Hmong child, her American doctors, and the collision of two cultures.* New York: Farrar, Straus, & Giroux.

Gollnick, D. M., & Chinn, P. C. (2001). *Multicultural education in a pluralistic society* (6th ed.). Upper Saddle River, NJ: Prentice-Hall.

Guralnick, M. J. (2008). International perspectives on early intervention: A search for common ground. *Journal of Early Intervention, 30*(2), 90–101.

Hanson, M. J. (2004). Ethnic, cultural, and language diversity in service settings. In E. W. Lynch & M. J. Hanson (Eds.), *Developing cross-cultural competence: A guide for working with children and their families* (pp. 3–18). Baltimore: Brookes.

Hanson, M. J., & Lynch, E. W. (2004). *Understanding families: Approaches to diversity, disability, and risk*. Baltimore: Brookes.

Hanson, M. J., Lynch, E. W., & Wayman, K. I. (1990). Honoring the cultural diversity of families when gathering data. *Topics in Early Childhood Special Education, 10*(1), 112–131.

Harry, B. (1992). Developing cultural self-awareness: The first step in values clarification for early service providers. *Topics in Early Childhood Special Education, 12*, 333–350.

Hernandez, D. J., Denton, N. A., & Macartney, S. E. (2008). Children in immigrant families: Looking to America's future. *Society for Research in Child Development, Social Policy Report, 22*(3), 3–11, 15, 17–22.

Klein, D. M., & White, J. M. (1996). *Family theories: An introduction*. Thousand Oaks, CA: Sage.

Lynch, E. W. (2004). Developing cross-cultural competence. In E. W. Lynch & M. J. Hanson (Eds.), *Developing cross-cultural competence: A guide for working with children and their families* (pp. 41–75). Baltimore: Brookes.

Lynch, E. W., & Hanson, M. J. (1993). Changing demographics: Implications for training in early intervention. *Infants and Young Children, 6*(1), 50–55.

Lynch, E. W., & Hanson, M. J. (2004). Implications for service providers. In E. W. Lynch & M. J. Hanson (Eds.), *Developing cross-cultural competence: A guide for working with children and their families* (pp. 449–466). Baltimore: Brookes.

Olson, S. (2001, April). The genetic archaeology of race. *The Atlantic Monthly*, 69–80.

Onaga, E. E., McKinney, K. G., & Pfaff, J. (2000). Lodge programs serving family functions for people with psychiatric disabilities. *Family Relations, 49*, 207–217.

Ronneau, J. P. (1999). Ordinary families—extraordinary caregiving. *Family Preservation Journal, 4*(1), 63–80.

Rorie, J. L., Paine, L. L., & Barger, M. K. (1996). Primary care for women: Cultural competence in primary care services. *Journal of Nurse Midwifery, 41*(2), 92–100.

Smith, E., & Sapp, W. (Eds.). (1996). *Plain talk about the Human Genome Project: A Tuskegee University conference on its promise and perils . . . and matters of race*. Tuskegee, AL: Tuskegee University Publications.

Turnbull, A. P., Summers, J. A., & Brotherson, M. J. (1984). *Working with families with disabled members: A family systems approach*. Lawrence: University of Kansas, Kansas Affiliated Facility.

Turnbull, A. P., Summers, J. A., Turnbull, R., Brotherson, M. J., Winton, P., Roberts, R., et al. (2007). Family supports ands services in early intervention: A bold vision. *Journal of Early Intervention, 29*(3), 187–206.

U.S. Census Bureau. (2008). *Language use and English-speaking ability: 2000*. Retrieved August 12, 2008, from *factfinder.census.gov/servlet/ACSSAFFPeople*.

Wayman, K. I., Lynch, E. W., & Hanson, M. J. (1990). Home-based early childhood services: Cultural sensitivity in a family systems approach. *Topics in Early Childhood Special Education, 10*(4), 65–66.

Checking the System for Cultural Competence

Question	Yes	Needs improvement	Not sure
1. Are the cultures, races, and languages spoken in the community mirrored in program staff and resources?			
2. Do program administrators and staff routinely interact with and seek the advice of community leaders or representative advisory boards?			
3. Is the program location accessible, approachable, and welcoming to families from diverse backgrounds?			
4. Are opportunities provided for families to be together if they choose?			
5. Are trained interpreters and translators available whenever needed?			
6. Are forms and other materials available in a variety of languages and formats?			
7. Is there a gathering place for families that is culturally inviting?			
8. Are there opportunities for families to develop new skills such as English-language classes and vocational training?			
9. Are staff members respectful to *all* families?			
10. Are home visits conducted to be comfortable for each family and are family traditions and beliefs respected?			

Checking Program Implementation for Cultural Competence

Question	We're doing well	We need to improve	We need more information
Finding our services (referral)			
1. Are our services listed and described in local newspapers and publications?			
2. Are our services listed and described in community gathering places such as churches, synagogues, temples, recreation centers, markets, and so on?			
3. Have community leaders been informed about our services, visited our programs, and been given print information?			
4. Is information about our services available in languages spoken by the community members, in print, and in alternative forms?			
5. Are referring programs and agencies in the community aware of our program and how to make referrals?			
6. Are initial contacts responded to promptly and in the family's preferred language?			
7. Do program staff members have backgrounds similar to families?			
Information gathering and assessment			
8. Are all processes and procedures explained in the family's preferred language with opportunities for follow-up and clarification?			
9. Are translators and interpreters trained and available when needed?			
10. Is one person responsible for information gathering and being with the family when other assessors are needed?			
11. Is culturally relevant information obtained nonintrusively?			

(cont.)

Question	We're doing well	We need to improve	We need more information
12. Are families encouraged to be involved in the assessment (e.g., holding the baby, playing with the child, eliciting language) in settings in which they are comfortable?			
Goal development			
13. Are families encouraged and assisted to develop goals?			
14. Are strategies for working on goals explained in the family's preferred language and demonstrated?			
15. Is information about each goal and strategy provided in the family's preferred language?			
Program implementation			
16. Are goals written to be meaningful within the family's cultural and sociocultural contexts?			
17. Are families asked about their comfort with implementation and their comments and reactions observed and acted upon?			
18. Do interventionists check with families to determine the continued relevance of goals?			
19. Are families given information about their child's progress and goal attainment in a format that is accessible to them?			
Program evaluation			
20. Is program evaluation systematic and ongoing?			
21. Are evaluation data collected from families in a culturally sensitive manner?			
22. Are community leaders and cultural mediators routinely used to gather evaluation information and provide suggestions for improvement?			
23. Are suggestions for improving the program's cultural competence acted upon?			

CHAPTER 7

A Primary-Coach Approach to Teaming and Supporting Families in Early Childhood Intervention

M'Lisa L. Shelden and Dathan D. Rush

In accordance with Part C of the Individuals with Disabilities Education Act (IDEA), the use of a primary service provider (PSP) has been identified as a recommended practice that can result in positive outcomes for young children with disabilities and their families, for discipline-specific professional organizations and for the early childhood intervention field at large (American Speech–Language–Hearing Association, 2008a, 2008b; Pilkington, 2006; Sandall, Hemmeter, Smith, & McLean, 2005; Vanderhoff, 2004; Woods, 2008; Workgroup on Principles and Practices in Natural Environments, 2007). The concept of the use of teams comprising individuals with a variety of expertise and knowledge in the field of early childhood has been a consistent component of educational legislation (Individuals with Disabilities Education Act Amendments, 20 U.S.C. § 1400 *et seq.*, 1997), recommended practice documents (Sandall et al., 2005), and theoretical and research literature (Antoniadis & Videlock, 1991; Briggs, 1997; Nash, 1990; Woodruff & McGonigel, 1988). The question before the field of early childhood intervention now is not *if* teams should be used, but *how* teams can be configured to work together effectively in a cost-effective manner to maximize benefits for young children with disabilities and their families. This chapter describes the characteristics of a primary-coach approach to teaming and assists programs and practitioners in implementing these practices. This approach is one particular application of the use of a primary service provider most typically associated with a transdisciplinary model of team interaction in early childhood intervention.

175

A primary-coach approach to teaming is implemented when an early intervention program is identified as a formal resource for early childhood intervention and family support, and the program employs or contracts with practitioners with diverse knowledge and experiences to support the child's parents and other primary care providers. Use of a primary-coach approach to teaming is not intended to limit a family's access to a range of supports and services, but instead to expand support for families of children with disabilities. The primary coach is the lead program resource and point of contact among other program staff, the family, and other care providers (i.e., the team). The primary coach mediates the family's and other care providers' skills and knowledge in relation to a range of priorities and needed or desired resources. The operational definition of a primary-coach approach to teaming is

> An established multidisciplinary team that meets regularly and selects one member as the primary coach who receives coaching from other team members, and uses coaching with parents and other care providers to support and strengthen their confidence and competence in promoting child learning and development and obtaining desired supports and resources in natural learning environments. (Shelden & Rush, 2007, p. 2)

The operational definition of a primary-coach approach to teaming differs from other approaches to teaming in which one practitioner serves as the primary liaison between the family and other team members (e.g., transdisciplinary) (Woodruff & McGonigel, 1988; York, Rainforth, & Giangreco, 1990) by an explicit focus on the type (i.e., coaching) and content (i.e., natural learning environment practices) of interactions between team members and their roles for promoting parent skills, knowledge, and attributions.

NATURAL LEARNING ENVIRONMENT PRACTICES

Natural learning environment practices are those practices that support parents and other care providers of children with disabilities in understanding the importance of everyday activities as the sources of children's learning opportunities. Dunst, Bruder, Trivette, Hamby, et al. (2001) defined an *activity setting* as a "situation-specific experience, opportunity, or event that involves a child's interaction with people, the physical environment, or both, which provides the contexts for a child to learn" (p. 70). Examples of activity settings include taking a bath, eating a meal, playing with pots and pans on the kitchen floor, swinging in a tire swing, feeding the dog, riding a bus downtown, reading a book before bedtime, and baking holiday cookies with Grandma. Natural learning environment practices also support parents and other care providers in recognizing and using child interests as a means for capitalizing on the abundant learning opportunities that exist in the lives of all children. *Interest-based learning* is defined as children's engagement in activities and with people and objects they find interesting, fun, exciting, and enjoyable (Dunst, Herter, & Shields, 2000; Raab, 2005). When a child is involved with something or someone that he or she finds interesting, research shows that the child will be engaged longer, thus yielding especially positive benefits related to child learning (Dunst et al., 2000; Raab, 2005).

Many practitioners have been trained to first identify delays in a child's skills and then teach parents strategies to "work on" skill development within a daily routine or activity setting. For example, if a child's language is delayed, a practitioner might teach the parent or caregiver a sign for "more" and direct the parent to use this sign to get the child to say or sign "more" throughout the day. In contrast, a practitioner who understands that child participation in activity settings *is* early childhood intervention spends time with the parent observing and identifying the child's interests and existing opportunities for interest expression during which the child has an inherent opportunity to learn and practice new skills. Consider an example in which a practitioner learns that a child loves to sit in his father's lap while the father reads the morning paper aloud (i.e., activity setting/child interest). The practitioner would encourage the father to continue this activity, discussing all the valuable learning opportunities afforded the child by participating in this interest-based activity setting on a regular basis. If the father is interested and willing, the practitioner could also discuss with him ways to involve the child further in the activity. The father might decide he would like to ask the child questions about pictures in the newspaper or simply comment on the pictures or advertisements. He might also want to experiment with allowing the child to help turn the pages, tell funny stories as if reading them from the paper, or ask the child to "read" from the paper. These are all examples of simple, responsive strategies the father could easily use to maintain the child's engagement in a fun and interesting activity that would not only lead to language development but also promote the child's social, cognitive, and motor skill development in a fun, interesting, and naturally occurring venue. The reader is referred to Dunst, Bruder, Trivette, and Hanby (2005, 2006) and Dunst, Bruder, Trivette, Hamby, et al. (2001) for additional information on natural learning environment practices.

COACHING FAMILIES

Coaching is an interactive process of reflection, information sharing, and action on the part of the primary coach and care providers, used to refine existing practices, develop new skills, and promote continuous self-assessment and learning on the part of the person being coached (e.g., Joyce & Showers, 1982; Kohler, McCullough, & Buchan, 1995; Morgan, Gustafson, Hudson, & Salzberg, 1992; Munro & Elliott, 1987; Peterson, Luze, Eshbaugh, Jeon, & Kantz, 2007; Rush, Shelden, & Hanft, 2003; Showers, 1985; Sparks, 1986; Tschantz & Vail, 2000). Coaching in early childhood may be conceptualized as a particular type of helpgiving practice within a capacity-building model to support family members and other care providers in using existing abilities and developing new skills to attain desired life circumstances (Dunst & Trivette, 1996; Dunst, Trivette, & LaPointe, 1992; Rappaport, 1981; Trivette & Dunst, 1998). Coaching of parents and other care providers by early childhood practitioners builds the capacity of family members to promote the child's learning and development.

Early childhood practitioners who use coaching facilitate a dynamic exchange of information, as well as model and practice new strategies based on the parent's intentions and current level of knowledge and skills necessary to promote the child's participation in family, community, and early childhood settings (Bruder & Dunst, 1999; Hanft, Rush, & Shelden, 2004). The role of the coach is to provide a supportive, nonhierarchical environment in which the parent and coach jointly examine and reflect on current practices, apply new skills and competencies with feedback, and address challenging situations. The coach's ultimate goal is ongoing performance in which the parent has the competence and confidence to engage in action, self-reflection, self-correction, and generalization of new skills and strategies to other situations as appropriate (Flaherty, 1999; Kinlaw, 1999).

Operational Definition of Coaching Practices

The definition of coaching developed and used by the authors focuses on the operationalization of the relationship between coaching practices and the intended consequences as well as the processes used to produce the observed changes (Dunst, Trivette, & Cutspec, 2002) and is based on a synthesis of research on coaching practices. Coaching may be defined as

> An adult learning strategy in which the coach promotes the learner's ability to reflect on his or her actions as a means to determine the effectiveness of an action or practice and develop a plan for refinement and use of the action in immediate and future situations. (Rush & Shelden, 2005, p. 3)

The following is a brief example of how a practitioner would engage a parent in a coaching interaction. Consider a situation in which the parent tells the practitioner that he would like for his child to sit in the cart at the grocery store so they can do their shopping and so his child can see what's going on around him. The practitioner asks what they've currently been doing during shopping and how well it has worked. The practitioner and father then brainstorm some ideas building on what the father has tried and plan to meet at the grocery store, for their next visit. The father places the child in the seat of the cart at the grocery store strapping him in as he and the practitioner had discussed. The child begins to fuss and cry and is also leaning to one side in the cart seat. The practitioner asks the father why he thinks the child might be crying. The father believes that the child's discomfort in the cart is what has upset him. The practitioner then asks what ideas the father might have to help the child sit straighter in the cart. The father tries repositioning the child, which does not seem to help and then decides to place the diaper bag next to the child to help straighten him up in the seat. The child also has a few of his favorite toys in the bag. As the father reaches to get out the toys, the practitioner asks the father, "How could we have your son be more active in choosing the toy?" The father indicates that he doesn't know what to do, and the practitioner models engaging the child in retrieving the toy from the bag. The practitioner asks the father how what she did compared to what he would normally do and he replied, "I didn't realize just choosing the toy would be something fun for him to do and look how he is playing with it instead of fussing." At the end of the shopping trip, the practitioner and father develop a plan that includes ways for the father to help the child sit upright in the grocery cart and ideas for additional interest-based activities for the child to do while the father shops for groceries.

Coaching Characteristics

The characteristics of a particular practice inform a practitioner of what to do to achieve the desired effect. An unpublished coaching research synthesis by the authors suggests that coaching has five practice characteristics that lead to intended outcomes: (1) joint planning, (2) observation, (3) action/practice, (4) reflection, and (5) feedback.

Joint Planning

Joint planning ensures the parent's active participation in the use of new knowledge and skills between coaching sessions. Joint planning occurs as a part of all coaching conversations, which typically involve discussion of what the parent agrees to do between coaching interactions to use the information discussed or skills that were practiced. For example, as a result of a coaching interaction between the parent and practitioner, the parent decides to get the high chair from the garage, clean it, and use it with her toddler during meals and snack times between visits.

Observation

Observation does not necessarily occur during every coaching conversation, but is used over the course of several coaching visits. Observation typically occurs by the practitioner directly observing an action on the part of the parent, which then provides an opportunity for later reflection and discussion (e.g., a practitioner observes a parent offering a child choices while getting dressed in the morning). Observation may also involve modeling by the practitioner for the parent. When the practitioner models for the parent, a three-step process is used that consists of preparation, modeling, and reflection. First, the practitioner discusses what he or she is going to do with the child and asks the parent to make specific observations while the modeling occurs. Second, the practitioner models for the parent by building upon what the parent is already doing and demonstrating additional strategies. Third, the practitioner prompts reflection by the parent regarding how his or her modeling matches the parent's intent, is similar to or different from what the parent typically does, and is consistent with what research informs us about child learning and what the parent wants or is willing to try based on the practitioner's modeling (e.g., following further discussion, the practitioner demonstrates offering the child choices while getting down on the child's level and making eye contact with the child).

Action/Practice

Actions are events or experiences that are planned or spontaneous, occur in the context of a real-life activity, and might take place when the coach is or is not present. The characteristic of action provides opportunities for the family member or care provider to use the information discussed during the coaching interaction. This type of active participation is a key characteristic of effective helpgiving and is an essential component for building the capacity of the person being coached. For example, between coaching conversations, when a parent and child get ready to go on a car trip, the parent lets the child know 15 minutes before the trip, allows the child enough time to maneuver his or her walker to the car, and provides just enough assistance to help the child climb up into the car and into his or her car seat.

Reflection

Reflection on the part of the person being coached is a critical characteristic that distinguishes coaching from consultation, supervision, and training. Reflection follows an observation or action and provides the parent an opportunity to analyze current strategies and refine his or her knowledge and skills. During reflection, the practitioner may ask the parent to describe what worked or did not work during observation or action, followed by generating alternatives and actions for continually improving his or her knowledge and skills.

Feedback

Feedback occurs after the parent has the opportunity to reflect on his or her observations, actions, or opportunity to practice new skills. Feedback includes statements by the practitioner that affirm the parent's reflections (e.g., "I understand what you are saying") or add information to deepen the parent's understanding of the topic. It also includes jointly developing new ideas and actions. When providing feedback, the coach shares information based on current research from his or her discipline-specific training, his or her own professional experience, and input from other team members. Sharing additional ideas for helping the child climb a slide following the parent's reflection on what he or she has tried and found to be either successful or unsuccessful is an example of informative feedback.

PRIMARY-COACH APPROACH TO TEAMING

Acknowledgment of the large amount of work contributed by teams in the workplace is common in business and industry (Cohen & Bailey, 1997; Hoegl & Gemuenden, 2001), education (Flowers, Mertens, & Mulhall, 1999), early childhood (Briggs, 1997; Woodruff & McGonigel, 1988) and health care contexts (Borrill et al., 2001; Borrill et al., 2002). The importance of teamwork in health care has also been documented in terms of benefits for health care workers (e.g., lower stress, higher retention rates, increased innovation by team members, increased job satisfaction) and recipients of services (e.g., lower mortality rates in hospitals; higher quality of care; improved cost-effectiveness) (Borrill et al., 2001, 2002). In a survey of U.S. organizations regarding team design variables and team effectiveness, more than 48% of respondents indicated the use of teams (Bell, 2004).

Effective Teaming Characteristics

Based on the work of Bell (2004) and others, succinctly put, effective teams consist of individuals who are agreeable; are conscientious; have high general mental ability; are competent in their area of expertise; are high in openness to experience and mental stability; like teamwork; and have been with the organization long enough to be socialized. For anyone who has participated as a team member over even a short period, these characteristics are not surprising. In fact, the simplicity of many of the characteristics may prove comforting to administrators and program coordinators across the country. As personnel are being considered to participate on identified teams, especially in terms of personal characteristics on the list (e.g., competence, conscientiousness, openness, mental stability, level of intelligence, agreeability, preference for teamwork), administrators could use a host of interview procedures and activities to determine a practitioner's "goodness of fit" for team membership.

The length of team membership and amount of time committed to the team are particularly relevant, considering the importance of consistent teams for children and their families in a primary-coach approach. This is particularly true for those states that use broker-type systems and vendors from a multitude of agencies where providers contract for an occasional hour in addition to their "real job" (Dunst & Bruder, 2006; Sloper, 2004; Sloper, Mukherjee, Beresford, Lightfoot, & Norris, 1999; Sloper & Turner, 1992). Team members should be assigned to a consistent team, so team members can identify readily who is on their team. The system must be able to support these teams in such a way as to minimize turnover, maximize involvement time, and promote long-term membership. Socialization and acculturation to the team and the employment of research-based practices is less likely to occur when team members rotate or change frequently. This socialization–acculturation effect described by Bell (2004) and others (Borrill et al., 2001, 2002) is one of the most positive benefits of implementing a primary-coach approach to teaming. The approach adds an inherent check and balance among team members, a heightened sense of responsibility, and programmatic accountability regarding the overall quality of supports and services for *all* families enrolled in the program. (See Appendix 7.1 at the end of this chapter.)

The following paragraphs summarize team task and structure factors related to implementation of a primary-coach approach to teaming.

• *Team task(s) should allow members to use a variety of skills, result in meaningful work, and have significant consequences for other people (Bell, 2004; Borrill et al., 2001; Hackman, 1987).* The team design literature identifies the importance of a team's task as a critical component regarding inherent motivation of the team, the commitment the team members have to accomplishing the task, and the development of a collective team identity in terms of completion of a job well-done. Within business and industry, the team task variable is discussed and studied as one that can be manipulated in an attempt to achieve higher motivation, commitment, and so on. In health and education, however, the argument can be made that motivation, commitment, satisfaction, and sense of responsibility are inherent to the task given to teams. For example, in early childhood intervention, teams are charged with and fully responsible for assisting family members and care providers in developing the confidence and competence individually needed (despite any and all challenges) to support the growth and development of the children in their care (IDEA, 1997).

• *The number of team members should be appropriate for the task (Bell, 2004; Larsson, 2000).* Bell (2004) stated that team size should be "just large enough to perform the task, thus each team member should bring a relatively unique set of task-relevant expertise to the team" (p. 22). Although the results of Bell's work depict no magical team size number, evidence continues to propose and is aligned with Hackman's (1987) early suggestions that teams with unnecessary members are not as productive as those teams with membership limited to those required to perform the task. Early childhood intervention programs are required by federal law to have a multidisciplinary team of practitioners available to families of children with disabilities (Individuals with Disabilities Education Act Amendments, 20 U.S.C. § 1400 *et seq.*, 1997), hence the requirement for teams implementing a primary-coach approach to secure participation of core disciplines essential to multidisciplinary representation (i.e., early childhood educator/special educator, occupational therapist, physical therapist, service coordinator, speech–language pathologist). While all core team members do not necessarily need to be reflected on the individualized family service plan (IFSP), these disciplines must be available to support the primary coach.

• *Teams should have some degree of self-managing abilities, because team self-management is related to enhanced team performance (Bell, 2004; Borrill et al., 2001; De Drue & West, 2001; Erez, LePine, & Elms, 2002).* Participation in team decision making is a critical factor in team innovation (i.e., pursuit, assimilation, and implementation of new ideas). Assignment of a team leader (or facilitator) is essential in most early childhood intervention programs, because of the documentation requirements associated with many team tasks, but involvement in team decision making is a critical factor in team productivity and innovation. Practically, appointment of a team leader who has skills in group facilitation will most likely result in a self-managing team having short decision times, self-implemented accountability strategies, and enhanced flexibility and efficiency. Teams with good self-management also need less supervisory or middle-management positions. Although implementing self-management is challenging, it appears to be beneficial for those in current state systems and programs, especially those using a brokered, independent provider system.

• *Teams should have a common planning time (Borrill et al., 2001, 2002; Flowers et al., 1999).* Common planning or meeting time for team members is essential to effective team functioning. In addition to providing team members with a predictable time for discussion, idea generation, questioning, and critical thinking, this regularly scheduled shared meeting time also contributes to the acculturation and socialization of the team identity and serves as the venue for the development of a heightened sense of accountability and commitment for completion of the task before the team.

Characteristics of a Primary-Coach Approach to Teaming

In light of the literature previously discussed and adhering to the evidence-based approach for documenting characteristics of specific practices described by Dunst et al. (2002), the following list depicts the characteristics of a primary-coach approach to teaming.

- An identified team of individuals from multiple disciplines having expertise in child development, family support, and coaching is assigned to each family in a program.
- One team member serves as primary coach to the care provider(s).
- The primary coach receives coaching from other team members through ongoing planned and spontaneous interactions.

Implementation Conditions

The following conditions are critical to effective implementation of the approach:

- All therapists and educators on the team must be available to serve as a primary coach.
- All team members attend regular team meetings for the purpose of colleague-to-colleague coaching. Coaching topics at team meetings are varied and include specific information for supporting team members in their role as a primary coach to the families in the program.
- The primary coach is selected according to desired outcomes of the family, the relationship between the coach and family, and the knowledge and availability of the coach and family.
- Visits by other team members should occur with the primary coach, at the same place and time whenever possible, to support the primary coach.
- The primary coach for a family should change as infrequently as possible. Justifiable reasons for changing the primary coach include a request by a family member or other care provider, or when a primary coach believes that even with coaching from other team members he or she is ineffective in supporting the care providers.

To provide a clear illustration of how a team would implement a primary-coach approach to teaming, the following section describes specific steps in how to go about this process.

Steps in Implementing a Primary-Coach Approach

- *Step 1: Identify a team.* One of the most exciting opportunities facing the early intervention system and the first step in moving to a primary-coach approach is establishing geographically based teams to support families and their children. Teams are not formed around individual children, but consist of representatives from a variety of disciplines who are assigned to provide supports within a given catchment area, geographic region, ZIP code, portion of a school district, and so on. A core team must minimally include one full-time equivalent of an early childhood educator or early childhood special educator, one occupational therapist, one physical therapist, and one speech–language pathologist for every 100 families, approximately. In Part C, the team must also include a service coordinator who is either one of the above core team members or a dedicated service coordinator depending on the state's guidelines for service coordination. If practitioners are also responsible for the role of service coordination or in situations that require extensive travel times, the number of families supported by the core team might need to be decreased. Other core team members might also include audiologists, nurses, dietitians, psychologists, social workers, teachers of children with vision or hearing impairments, mobility specialists, physicians, assistive technology specialists, and so on. Custodial family members are always part of their child's team. Circumstances specific to a particular child may require additional team members such as Head Start and Early Head Start teachers, Parents as Teachers home visitors, child care providers, and any other individuals parents deem important in the life of the child.

Individuals serving in a support role such as aides, assistants, and paraprofessionals are not members of the core team. Based on a scarcity model of practitioner availability, assistants typically work under the direction of one of the aforementioned core team members for the sole purpose of providing more of a specific traditional therapy regimen to the child (e.g., a physical therapist assistant goes to the child's home for practice walking with a walker). A primary-coach approach to teaming uses natural learning environment practices to promote parent competence and confidence in using everyday activities as opportunities for child learning. This approach requires the expertise of and accessibility to the supervising therapist or educator to maximize just-in-time learning opportunities and continue the ongoing conversation to coach the parent or other care provider rather than using an assistant to implement an approved exercise program or standard set of activities. A limited number of state licensure laws allow autonomous practice of therapy assistants. In these rare circumstances, assistants could be considered as members of a core team, but this is not recommended practice, and the assistant should never be substituted for a licensed therapist.

The team must have a designated leader who is minimally responsible for facilitating the team meetings and whose role is also to prepare the team meeting agenda, guide the discussion during the team meeting, and prepare the team minutes. Other responsibilities of the team leader might include coordinating referrals, assigning evaluators, reviewing documentation, and so on. The team leader might be a program administrator, service coordinator, or other team member. For consistency, the team leader role should be filled by the same person and not rotated among team members (Borrill et al., 2001; Erez et al., 2002). Appointment of a team leader based on title alone should be avoided, if possible, and maximizing participative decision making for all team members will result in better team performance (Bell, 2004). The team leader, whether appointed or allowed to emerge over time, must, however, have skills in group facilitation and demonstrate organizational skills and the ability to manage the regularly scheduled team meetings required by use of this approach.

The purpose of the team meeting when using a primary-coach approach is to share information among team members as families move through the early intervention process and for primary coaches to receive coaching from their team members. All team members attend regular (weekly) team meetings for colleague-to-colleague coaching. Families are aware when their primary coach will be going to the regular team meetings to seek coaching from other team members relative to their discussions. This need for coaching comes about as a result of a conversation between the primary coach and the family or other care provider. No decisions are made at meetings without the family; rather the primary coach gathers additional information to give to the parent. When the family wants to meet with the entire team, these meetings should be held at a time and location convenient for the family.

The steps for moving to a team-based approach for providing early childhood intervention supports are as follows:

1. Determine the distribution of eligible families across the catchment area.
2. Identify the geographic area the team is to cover (i.e., counties, ZIP codes, school districts), based on family distribution.
3. Determine the number of teams necessary to cover each designated area.
4. Assign available practitioners to teams, beginning with those who can give the most time to the program.
5. Develop a mechanism to compensate team members for team meeting time.

- *Step 2: Gather information.* The initial conversations with the family are critical. During these conversations, the person functioning in the service coordination role engages the parent in a conversation about family, community, and early childhood program activity settings and child interests. Activity settings and interests serve as the foundation on which the early intervention team and family support the child's participation (Dunst, Bruder, Trivette, Hamby, et al., 2001; Göncü, 1999). Child participation in meaningful activities provides opportunities for the child to practice existing skills and learn new abilities (Dunst, Bruder, Trivette, Raab, & McLean, 2001). Without a clear understanding of activities important to the family as well as those that are of high interest to the child, the tendency of most practitioners is to identify skills to be taught, strategies to use to teach those skills, and then activities in which the strategies can be placed. Within this traditional approach, the practitioner and parent focus on the desired skills and strategies rather than on supporting the child's participation in the activity, which actually might require the identification of a range of strategies. The focus, therefore, remains on the child's participation in the activity, which provides opportunities for skill development and practice.

Assessment is the process used to analyze the child's current level of participation within the identified activity settings as well as the degree of parent or care provider responsiveness to the child. As part of the assessment process, the practitioner and parent may try a variety of strategies to assist the child to participate in activities that he or she wants and needs to do more fully. For example, if the child needs to be able to get on the toilet, the practitioner and parent may try a number of different ways of assisting the child to discover the most viable option. As opposed to evaluation, which determines a child's initial and ongoing eligibility, assessment is an ongoing process that when done well, is difficult to differentiate from intervention.

- *Step 3: Develop participation-based IFSP outcomes.* IFSP outcomes should be functional and based on family and care provider priorities and can be child- or family-focused (Able-Boone, 1993; Boone, McBride, Swann, Moore, & Drew, 1998; Rosin et al., 1996). When team members obtain information about child participation in current and desired activity settings as the sources of children's learning opportunities, IFSP outcomes naturally flow from the conversations with parents and other care providers. Because the conversation is contextualized around child participation in current and desired activities rather than limited to identification of deficits and parental concerns, parents know what they want the child's participation to look like within those activities, which become potential outcomes on the IFSP. For example, if presently the mother must carry the child around the home with her or lay down the child in order to do her household chores, but she has expressed a desire to have the child play with toys to entertain him- or herself while she does her chores, then this would be the outcome. In contrast, since the child is unable to sit independently, a more traditional skill-based outcome would be for the child to sit independently for at least 5 minutes.

Figure 7.1 provides additional examples of participation-based, functional IFSP outcomes for implementation by a primary coach and parents. (See the "Taylor Family Case Example" later in this chapter for additional examples of participation-based, functional IFSP outcomes. See also R. A. McWilliam, Chapter 2, this volume, on the Routines-Based Interview.)

• *Step 4: Identify the primary coach.* All team members should be competent and confident in their own discipline, child development, parenting supports, natural learning environment practices, and coaching. Any core team member may be the primary coach, with the exception of the service coordinator in systems that use a dedicated service coordinator. Although a dedicated service coordinator may use a coaching style of interaction, he or she would not be the primary coach. The person selected to be primary coach is the member of the team who is the best possible match for a family and may be selected based on four criteria: IFSP

Child-focused IFSP outcomes	Family-focused IFSP outcomes
Jimmy will have fun playing with his toys and his brother while positioned comfortably throughout the day.	Dana and Barbara will learn a variety of new strategies, including positioning, which they can use to make Jimmy's play time more enjoyable for him.
Mark will gain weight so that he will be consistently healthy.	Dorothy and Roger will ensure that Mark has daily access to the nutritional and medical resources he needs in his home and community so that he will be consistently healthy.
Sally will feed herself using her fingers and a spoon during mealtime and snack time daily.	Miss Fern (at child care) will feel comfortable letting Sally learn how to feed herself.
LaKeisha will put on her own shirt and pull up her pants by her third birthday.	LaKeisha's grandma will know strategies for helping LaKeisha dress herself without a fuss.
Robbie will enjoy his favorite activities of book reading and having snacks while riding in the grocery cart during shopping trips with his father.	Robert Sr. and Robbie will complete their grocery shopping trips within 30 minutes with Robbie being content and remaining in the grocery cart.

FIGURE 7.1. Sample individualized family service plan (IFSP) outcomes.

outcomes; relationship with the parent, care provider, or other primary learner; special knowledge of the coach; and availability of the team member to be a family's primary coach.

IFSP outcomes are priorities set by the family. Since outcomes should be functional and discipline-free, taking all of the outcomes on the IFSP into consideration, the best primary coach would be the team member who can support the parents or other primary learner(s) in accomplishing them. For example, if the IFSP contains only one outcome and it is "the child will eat with the family at mealtime," then the primary coach should be the team member who excels at supporting families around mealtime. If the only outcome on the IFSP is "the family will have happy car rides when taking the children to and from school," then the person on the team selected to be the primary coach should be the team member who is the very best at supporting families in happy car rides. If both outcomes are on the IFSP, then the team would select the team member best suited to assist the family in accomplishing both outcomes. The primary coach would then identify other supports needed from the team in assisting him or her in helping the family accomplish these outcomes.

Another criterion used to select the primary coach is the relationship a member of the team may already have with a family member or care provider. For example, if a family has an older child who participated in the program, then the person who worked most closely with the parent or care provider at that time may be the best choice to become the primary coach. In this situation, the relationship may already be established, and the primary coach and family members already know how to work with one another. Since the primary coach is competent and confident in child development, parenting supports, and coaching, and also knows when to seek support from other members of the team, the team member with a preexisting relationship may be the best choice for primary coach.

A match between the specialized knowledge of a team member and the priorities of the family is another criterion that may be used to select the primary coach. Typically, new teams most often use this criterion for selecting the primary coach. Initially, they choose the person from the discipline most closely associated with the family's priorities. As an example, if the family wants their child to be able to participate in a conversation with them, the team might select the speech–language pathologist to be the primary coach. As the team works together over time and comes to know one another for their individual knowledge and experiences as well as discipline-specific knowledge, the team becomes more comfortable in selecting the primary coach based on his or her professional expertise as well as life experiences, rather than strictly on the discipline of the practitioner. In the example above, the early childhood special education teacher or the early childhood educator may be equally as competent as the speech–language pathologist to provide this type of support to the family as primary coach depending on the specific circumstances or underlying causes of the limitations in the child's participation. When a team member has particular knowledge, expertise, or skills that might be useful to a family, that individual may be the best team member to serve as primary coach.

Another criterion for selecting the primary coach is availability. If a team member's schedule is essentially full and he or she cannot take another family into his or her caseload, then he or she may not be available to be the primary coach. However, if he or she is the best and only person who should be the primary coach for the family, then the team will have to determine whether some adjustments can be made to enable him or her to provide support to the new family. If the best person on the team cannot be made available to the family and no other team member has the knowledge and skills necessary to support the family, the team may have to identify a resource outside the team. Rarely does a team have to seek outside resources as adjustments can usually be made within the team for the family to have the best possible primary coach.

One of the purposes in having a primary coach is for the family to establish and maintain an ongoing working relationship with a single team member to minimize any negative consequences of having multiple and or changing practitioners. As a result, the primary coach rarely changes. The primary coach does not change when IFSP outcomes change, when primary learners change, or when the primary coach may need specific supports from other team members. The primary coach should change if the family does not like the manner or style of the primary coach, the family specifically requests a change, or the primary coach continually needs another team member on joint visits because of his or her lack of knowledge and skill.

Once the primary coach is selected, the frequency, intensity, and duration of the supports must be specified. Previous methods for determining frequency and intensity of services have been based on severity of the child's disability, age of the child, availability of openings in the practitioners' schedules, socioeconomic status of the family, education level of the primary care provider, number of years in therapy, practitioner judgment of the parents' ability to follow through with a home program, match of cognitive level of child to other areas of developmental status (i.e., cognitive referencing) and third-party reimbursement caps (Atwater, McEwen, & McMillan, 1982; Borkowski & Wessman, 1994; Carr, 1989; Cole, Dale, & Mills, 1990; Cole & Mills, 1997; Cole, Mills, & Harris, 1991; Dunst & Trivette, 2002; Farley, Sarracino, & Howard, 1991; Krassowski & Plante, 1997; Notari, Cole, & Mills, 1992). None of these methods have been found to be effective ways to determine need, frequency, intensity, or duration of service.

Regardless of the scheduling methods previously used, determining the frequency, intensity, and duration of visits when using a primary-coach approach to teaming is a completely different process. This process is part of the joint planning conversation with the parents and other care providers determined by the desired level of support needed by the parents to promote their competence and confidence in using natural learning opportunities to foster their child's learning and development. For example, the conversation with the parents would be based on a summary of the visit, followed by asking the parents how much time they need to implement the plan discussed and when they would need and prefer the practitioner to return. To operationalize this just-in-time method of support, the flexibility of the IFSP must be maximized to capture the estimated amount of support necessary to assist the family in achieving the IFSP outcomes. A sample frequency and intensity statement might be: "Between January 3 and April 3, 2006, twenty 1-hour visits will occur in the home and child care settings." The IFSP is a promise between the program and the family; therefore, adjustments may be necessary to increase or decrease the number of visits in order to meet the identified outcomes within the established time period.

• *Step 5: Use natural learning environment practices to build the capacity of care providers to promote child learning.* Using the information regarding interest-based activity settings and the important people in the child's life obtained in Step 2, the primary coach uses coaching as the adult learning strategy with the parents and other care providers to build their capacity to promote the child's learning and development. Interactions between the coach and care provider minimally include an opportunity for the parent or other care provider to reflect on what he or she is doing to support the child in accomplishing the desired priorities and for the coach and care provider to generate other strategies or ideas to try within the context of child interest-based activities. For example, consider a scenario in which the speech–language pathologist (SLP) is the primary coach for a child whose family's priority is for the child to play with his or her brother and sister in the backyard. The parents and siblings of the child need support around how to use the child's interests to maximize playing happily and safely together outside. Some of the strategies used by the family will be targeting their responsiveness regarding the child's communication. Other strategies involve the parents' use of behavioral supports during the playtime and techniques for assisting the child to keep up with the siblings as they move about the backyard. During visits, the SLP observes the family's use of jointly identified strategies to promote the child's participation in backyard play. The SLP (primary coach) also provides feedback on the family's implementation of the plan, demonstrates alternative uses of particular strategies, observes additional demonstrations by the family to check for understanding, and jointly plans the next steps that will happen in between visits.

Taylor Family Case Example

The following case example was designed to depict practical application of the information provided in this chapter.

Consider an early intervention team using a primary coach approach to teaming that has just received a referral from a family new to the local area. The family is currently living in an apartment in a suburb of a large metropolitan area. The Taylor family consists of Debra (mother), Wayne (father), and Felicity, their 2-year-old daughter. Debra and Wayne Taylor have expressed interest in receiving assistance from the early intervention program to support Felicity's growth and development. The Taylor family likes to watch television as their favorite family pastime, and they have a new puppy that lives indoors. Wayne is in the United States Air Force stationed at a base approximately 10 miles from their apartment, and Debra stays home full time to care for Felicity. Felicity was diagnosed with cerebral palsy shortly after birth. According to Debra, Felicity likes being held by her mom, is very interested in the new puppy, and doesn't like to eat. Felicity weighs 20 pounds and her parents and physician are worried about her ability to gain weight. She drinks from a bottle but vomits most of the formula soon after eating. She is held for eating and is unable to join the family at the table for dinner. She requires support to sit or use her hands and is unable to move around the apartment independently. Felicity indicates her happiness by smiling, and sadness by crying.

After the Taylor family was referred to the early intervention program, the referral coordinator assigned the family to the team responsible for providing support in the Taylor family's ZIP code area. One of the team service coordinators was assigned to the family and scheduled a meeting with them to discuss their priorities and questions and begin the initial assessment process of identifying the family's activity settings and interests. The priorities of the Taylor family were then presented at the weekly team meeting. The team quickly recognized that Felicity was obviously eligible and was able to document eligibility based on medical records. The team then planned further assessment by the person on the team with expertise in feeding and eating issues. In this case, the occupational therapist (OT) was selected on the basis of the family's prevailing priority of helping Felicity gain weight. The lead practitioners prepared a team report that summarized the priorities, interests, and activity settings of the family and information that documented Felicity's eligibility for the early intervention program. This information was then forwarded to Felicity's physician with permission of the parents. The next step was a joint meeting among the family and other team members to write the IFSP. They identified outcomes that addressed the Taylor family's priorities and would promote Felicity's participation in family activities and routines (e.g., joining the family at the table for dinner, bathing, watching TV, going to the grocery store, visiting the apartment complex playground). At the IFSP meeting, held in July, the team identified the following outcomes:

1. Felicity will gain 5 pounds over the next 6 months.
2. Felicity will join the family at the dinner table and eat strained food while seated in her high chair by Thanksgiving.
3. Debra will learn strategies to help her be comfortable having fun and playing with Felicity.
4. Debra and Wayne will learn new ways to expect Felicity to let them know what she wants, likes, and doesn't like to do by Christmas.

Note that specific support decisions were made after the development and prioritization of IFSP outcomes, not before.) The family and therapists next decided the primary coach would be the team's OT, who up to this point had the most contact with the family and also felt comfortable supporting the family around the identified outcomes on the IFSP. The frequency of visits by the primary coach was then decided based on the level of support Debra and Wayne desired. The team decided that between July 5 and January 5, the primary coach (OT) would visit the Taylor home for thirty-four, 1-hour visits. Additionally, between July 5 and August 5, the physical therapist would visit the Taylor home *with the primary coach* for eight, 1-hour visits. Weekly, all other team members were available for coaching support at the regularly scheduled team meetings. The team felt it was important for the frequency and intensity of services to be higher, initially, and then to decrease as priorities were achieved and Wayne's and Debra's confidence in supporting Felicity increased. The primary coach (OT) also knew that he would need initial support from the physical therapist for several visits to assist with provision and implementation of assistive technology (e.g., high chair seat insert, foot splints, bath chair, and other aids) to occur in the Taylor home. The OT also received ongoing coaching from the other team members to assist him in strengthening the ability of Debra and Wayne to help their daughter gain weight and join them at the dinner table at mealtime to learn responsive teaching strategies that assist them in parenting. The initial plan was tentative, but looked like the following:

Primary Coach Visits

Weeks 1–2 = six 1-hour visits
Weeks 3–4 = four 1-hour visits
Months 2–3 = twelve 1-hour visits
Months 4–6 = twelve 1-hour visits

Joint Visits by Physical Therapist with Primary Coach

Weeks 1–4 = eight 1-hour visits

The role of the primary coach in this approach was to focus on supporting Debra and Wayne in addressing their priorities and maximizing Felicity's participation in current and desired activity settings. The primary coach would use coaching strategies and natural learning environment practices to support the Taylor family's understanding of how Felicity's everyday learning experiences afforded many opportunities for supporting her growth and development. The focus of the primary coach would not only be on what happened during his scheduled visits, but what happened when he wasn't present as well. For example, addressing the priority of having Felicity join the family at the dinner table and eat strained foods, the primary coach (OT) assisted the family in considering seating options (i.e., car seat, high chair, and booster seat) and different types of spoons to try for introducing foods. The primary coach also helped the family recognize opportunities when Felicity initiated communication with them during mealtime.

In the primary-coach approach to teaming, the Taylor family had access to an entire team of professionals, but was not constrained by the time it took for separate visits and was able to experience the benefits of using everyday situations as powerful learning opportunities that inherently had therapeutic benefits. The Taylor family met regularly with their primary coach who received coaching from other team members and supported the Taylor family's use of everyday experiences based on child and family interests as learning opportunities for Felicity. The responsibility of coordinating communication among team members was placed on the primary coach through ongoing interaction with the parents and receipt of coaching from other team members through weekly team meetings and joint visits.

CHALLENGES TO THE FIELD

Although use of a coaching interaction style, natural learning environment practices, and a primary-coach approach to teaming are consistent with how to support families in promoting their children's learning, a number of barriers and challenges to using these approaches exist for programs and systems that must either be minimized or eliminated entirely. Regardless of the model a program chooses to use, funding is a major barrier for implementation of early intervention supports and services. The first challenge to all early intervention programs is to maximize efficiency of resources through appropriate use of all available funding streams (i.e., federal Part C dollars, state-allocated funds, third-party reimbursement) without allowing traditional views of payment to drive the decisions about services and supports for eligible children and their families. The issue of the cost of a primary-coach approach to teaming has yet to be empirically determined, although several studies have suggested that choosing a primary provider as the liaison from a program to support families and their children may prove to be more cost-efficient (Barnett & Escobar, 1990; Barnett, Escobar, & Ravsten, 1988; Borrill et al., 2001; Eiserman, McCoun, & Escobar, 1990; Tarr & Barnett, 2001; Warfield, 1995).

In a primary-coach approach to teaming all team members are at the table (i.e., team meeting), and decisions are based on what supports are needed to assist care providers in enhancing their abilities to be confident and competent in supporting the growth and development of the children in their care. When contractors of the early intervention program are required to submit third-party billing, individually, as payment for their early intervention services, the issue of payment continues to stay at the forefront of the practitioner's involvement in the program. To shift the focus from what practitioners can be reimbursed by third-party payers to implementing supports needed by the family to achieve functional, meaningful, and participation-based IFSP outcomes, early intervention programs should consider central billing support for practitioners (contracted and employee), alternative payment sources for visits not billable to third-party payers, employment of practitioners versus extensive or exclusive use of contracting with providers, and use of quality assurance measures so that program administration are aware of the practices being implemented on behalf of the early intervention program.

Second, to implement a primary-coach approach to teaming effectively, support by program leadership is required. Program administrators must be knowledgeable about evidence-based practices and hold practitioners accountable for staying current, not only in their own discipline, but in the field of early childhood intervention as well. Practitioners who are either directly employed by a program or are on contract serve as agents of the program and thereby should be held accountable for providing supports in a way that is consistent with research-based practices in the field, rather than using practices tied to preference or experience alone. Further, program administrators should ensure that program policies and procedures promote the use of practices that stem from current research and work to create a culture for reflection on practices to promote ongoing interdisciplinary learning.

Third, programs that use lists of approved providers from which families select practitioners to meet their needs or other forms of brokered services create a daunting challenge to the use of any type of teaming approach, but especially a primary-coach approach to teaming. Within these models, families most often rely on their service coordinator for guidance in choosing a provider. True teams are not formed, but rather families receive services from a group of practitioners who may or may not include multiple disciplinary perspectives, are not required to communicate with one another, meet only for the purposes of the IFSP meeting (if even then), and are focused only on the deficits they identify from their discipline-specific viewpoint. These groups of practitioners, especially in more populated areas, generally do not work together over time and with the same children, but rather are serendipitously formed by either the service coordinator or the family's selections from a list of available providers.

Frequently, practitioners and service coordinators raise concern that assigning a designated team to families rather than letting families select from a matrix or list restricts family choice. Selecting from a matrix may actually restrict the family to the limited disciplines selected rather than providing the family immediate and ongoing access to a team of individuals from multiple disciplines. Within a primary-coach approach to teaming, families participate in the decision of who the primary coach is going to be and why, thereby making an informed decision about their child's and family's services and supports. Additionally, if parents find they are unhappy with their choice, they may request a change of primary coach.

Fourth, in order to function effectively, teams must have regularly scheduled meeting time, to provide coaching to each other, receive coaching, plan joint visits, and plan their participation in evaluations, assessments, and IFSP meetings. In this way all team members' time is used more efficiently, and service coordinators can implement resource-based supports with families. In addition to better communication, team meetings offer opportunities for team members to hold one another mutually accountable for the use of up-to-date practices resulting in effective supports for children and families. Programs that use contracted practitioners must have mechanisms in place to pay all team members to attend these meetings. Furthermore, all core team members must be present for the team meeting. Inability of one or more team members to participate, either for lack of payment or time, hampers effective team functioning and forces team members to use a consultative model at best.

Fifth, understanding how to use a team-based approach in early childhood intervention should begin at the preservice level. Preservice educators should teach practices grounded in current research to ensure that students are good at what we know works. Preservice educators should model evidence-based teaching practices as well. Sound conceptual and theoretical frameworks must be provided when teaching promising practices. Critically important, preservice students should have interdisciplinary learning experiences in which they become familiar with other disciplines and how to work together to maximize the benefits to children with disabilities and their families. All field work experiences should be followed by critical analysis between students, faculty members, and field work supervisors regarding how what they observed and were asked to do was congruent with what we know from research.

Sixth, teams must have access to a full complement of disciplines to practice in a manner consistent with the characteristics of a primary-coach approach to teaming. A full complement would minimally include an early childhood educator/early childhood special educator, an OT, a physical therapist, a speech–language pathologist, and a service coordinator, if the system uses a dedicated service coordination model. In rural and remote areas, fulfilling this requirement can be particularly difficult when a perceived shortage of therapists or educators exists. In these circumstances, the most effective strategy is to recruit and hire a core team. When this is not an option, programs and systems must have mechanisms in place for providing financial and other incentives to recruit and retain qualified team members on a contractual basis. In addition, the use of technology may be necessary to link the team together for meetings, one-on-one coaching opportunities, and joint visits.

Seventh, developing the IFSP is a key component of how supports and services are provided for young children and their families. The IFSP process has been a topic of substantial rhetoric in early childhood literature, including information that summarizes problems with the process and delineates characteristics of practices that, when present, notably improve the process (Bailey, Winton, Rouse, & Turnbull, 1990; Dunst, Bruder, Trivette, Raab, & McLean, 1998; McWilliam, Ferguson, Harbin, Porter, & Vaderviere, 1998). Features of the IFSP process that are family-centered and facilitate the development of a meaningful IFSP include initiating the IFSP process on the first contact with the family to identify care provider priorities; involving all of the parties affected by the IFSP (i.e., parents, extended family members, child care providers); assessing the child within the context of real-life activities related to the care providers' priorities; and designing supports and services *after* the IFSP outcomes are identified. Outcome selection should focus on supporting adults in feeling confident and competent in promoting the child's participation in activity settings important to the child, family, and other care providers.

One challenge faced by many early intervention programs is the use of child-focused, discriminative evaluation procedures to determine services needed versus (1) the use of the evaluation methods to determine eligibility into the program, and (2) functional assessment strategies to develop participation-based outcomes to be used by the primary coach and care providers. In a primary-coach approach to teaming, coordinating multiple providers is streamlined because the team schedules the evaluation and assessment based on the families priorities within the context of everyday activities. Having multiple providers conduct separate evaluations typically leads to services delineated on the IFSP requiring that multiple service providers "work on" discipline-specific, deficit-based outcomes (i.e., gross motor outcomes written and addressed by a physical therapist, fine motor outcomes written and addressed by an OT). To promote efficiency and accountability, the Part C system is challenged to implement processes that deemphasize evaluation, reemphasize and support assessments of child participation within activity settings, and ensure that identified teams are responsible to families within a specific geographic area from initial contact through transition.

CONCLUSION

The federal regulations clearly delineate the involvement of teams comprising individuals from multiple disciplines in the design of delivery of early childhood supports and services, and discipline-specific professional organizations have followed suit in providing guidelines relative to functioning as a primary coach in early intervention. This chapter has focused on the use of a primary-coach approach to teaming to support young children with disabilities and their families in natural learning environments. The primary coach is responsible for implementing natural learning environment practices using a coaching style of interaction for enhancing the knowledge and skills of the primary care provider(s) to promote positive family functioning, maximize opportunities for child learning, and facilitate expansion of existing development-enhancing experiences within the context of everyday life. Early intervention programs must diligently use practices that are effective and efficient for children with disabilities and their families as well as consistent with how young children learn.

REFERENCES

Able-Boone, H. (1993). Family participation in the IFSP process: Family or professional driven? *Infant–Toddler Intervention, 3,* 63–71.

American Speech–Language–Hearing Association. (2008a). *Roles and responsibilities of speech–language pathologists in early intervention: Guidelines*. Rockville, MD: Author. Available from *www.asha.org/policy*.

American Speech–Language–Hearing Association. (2008b). *Roles and responsibilities of speech–language pathologists in early intervention: Technical report*. Rockville, MD: Author. Available from *www.asha.org/policy*.

Antoniadis, A., & Videlock, J. L. (1991). In search of teamwork: A transactional approach to team functioning. *Infant–Toddler Intervention, 1*, 157–167.

Atwater, S. W., McEwen, I. R., & McMillan, J. (1982). Assessment of the reliability of pediatric screening: A tool for occupational and physical therapists. *Physical Therapy, 62*(9), 1265–1268.

Bailey, D. B., Winton, P. J., Rouse, L., & Turnbull, A. P. (1990). Family goals in infant intervention: Analysis and issues. *Journal of Early Intervention, 14*, 15–26.

Barnett, W. S., & Escobar, C. M. (1990). Economic costs and benefits of early intervention In S. J. Meisels & J. P. Shonkoff (Eds.), *Handbook of early childhood intervention* (pp. 560–582).

Barnett, W. S., Escobar, C. M., & Ravsten, M. T. (1988). Parent and clinic early intervention for children with language handicaps: A cost-effectiveness analysis. *Journal of the Division for Early Childhood, 12*, 290–298.

Bell, S. T. (2004). *Setting the stage for effective teams: A meta-analysis of team design variables and team effectiveness*. Unpublished doctoral dissertation, Texas A & M University, College Station.

Boone, H. A., McBride, S. L., Swann, D., Moore, S., & Drew, B. S. (1998). IFSP practices in two states: Implications for practice. *Infants and Young Children, 10*(4), 36–45.

Borkowski, M. A., & Wessman, H. C. (1994). Determination of eligibility for physical therapy in the public school setting. *Pediatric Physical Therapy, 6*(2), 61–67.

Borrill, C. S., Carletta, A. J., Dawson, J. F., Garrod, S., Rees, A., Richards, A., et al. (2001). The effectiveness of health care teams in the National Health Service. Birmingham, UK: Aston Centre for Health Service Organizational Research, University of Aston.

Borrill, C. S., West, M. A., Dawson, J., Shapiro, D., Rees, A., Richards, A., et al. (2002). Team working and effectiveness in health care. Birmingham, UK: Aston Centre for Health Service Organisation Research, University of Aston.

Briggs, M. H. (1997). *Building early intervention teams: Working together for children and families*. Gaithersburg, MD: Aspen.

Bruder, M. B., & Dunst, C. J. (1999). Expanding learning opportunities for infants and toddlers in natural environments: A chance to reconceptualize early intervention. *Zero to Three, 20*(3), 34–36.

Carr, S. H. (1989). Louisiana's criteria of eligibility for occupational therapy services in the public school system. *American Journal of Occupational Therapy, 43*(8), 503.

Cohen, S. G., & Bailey, D. E. (1997). What makes teams work: Group effectiveness research from the shop floor to the executive suite. *Journal of Management, 23*, 239–291.

Cole, K. N., Dale, P. S., & Mills, P. E. (1990). Defining language delay in young children by cognitive referencing: Are we saying more than we know? *Applied Psycholinguistics, 11*, 291–302.

Cole, K. N., & Mills, P. E. (1997). Agreement of language intervention triage profiles. *Topics in Early Childhood Special Education, 17*, 119–130.

Cole, K. N., Mills, P. E., & Harris, S. R. (1991). Retrospective analysis of physical and occupational therapy progress in young children: An examination of cognitive referencing. *Pediatric Physical Therapy, 3,* 185–189.

De Drue, C. K. W., & West, M. A. (2001). Minority dissent and team innovation: The importance of participation in decision making. *Journal of Applied Psychology, 86*(4), 1191–1201.

Dunst, C. J., & Bruder, M. B. (2006). Early intervention service coordination models and service coordinator practices. *Journal of Early Intervention, 28,* 155–165.

Dunst, C. J., Bruder, M. B., Trivette, C. M., & Hamby, D. W. (2005). Young children's natural learning environments: Contrasting approaches to early childhood intervention indicate differential learning opportunities. *Psychological Reports, 96,* 231–234.

Dunst, C. J., Bruder, M. B., Trivette, C. M., & Hamby, D. W. (2006). Everyday activity settings, natural learning environments, and early intervention practices. *Journal of Policy and Practice in Intellectual Disabilities, 3,* 3–10.

Dunst, C. J., Bruder, M. B., Trivette, C. M., Hamby, D., Raab, M., & McLean, M. (2001). Characteristics and consequences of everyday natural learning opportunities. *Topics in Early Childhood Special Education, 21,* 68–92.

Dunst, C. J., Bruder, M. B., Trivette, C. M., Raab, M., & McLean, M. (1998, May). *Increasing children's learning opportunities through families and communities early childhood research institute: Year 2 progress report.* Asheville, NC: Orelena Hawks Puckett Institute.

Dunst, C. J., Bruder, M. B., Trivette, C. M., Raab, M., & McLean, M. (2001). Natural learning opportunities for infants, toddlers, and preschoolers. *Young Exceptional Children, 4*(3), 18–25 (Erratum in Vol. 4(4), 25).

Dunst, C. J., Herter, S., & Shields, H. (2000). Interest-based natural learning opportunities. In S. Sandall & M. Ostrosky (Eds.), *Natural Environments and Inclusion* (Young Exceptional Children Monograph Series No. 2) (pp. 37–48). Longmont, CO: Sopris West.

Dunst, C. J., & Trivette, C. M. (1996). Empowerment, effective helpgiving practices and family-centered care. *Pediatric Nursing, 22,* 334–337, 343.

Dunst, C. J., & Trivette, C. M. (2002). *Family resource center information and support scale.* Asheville, NC: Winterberry Press.

Dunst, C. J., Trivette, C. M., & Cutspec, P. A. (2002). Toward an operational definition of evidence-based practices. *Centerscope, 1*(1), 1–10. Available at *www.researchtopractice. info/centerscopes/centerscope_vol1_no1.pdf.*

Dunst, C. J., Trivette, C. M., & LaPointe, N. (1992). Toward clarification of the meaning and key elements of empowerment. *Family Science Review, 5,* 111–130.

Eiserman, W. D., McCoun, M., & Escobar, C. M. (1990). A cost-effectiveness analysis of two alternative program models for serving speech-disordered preschoolers. *Journal of Early Intervention, 14,* 297–317.

Erez, A., LePine, J. A., & Elms, H. (2002). Effects of rotated leadership and peer evaluation on the functioning and effectiveness of self-managed teams: A quasi-experiment. *Personnel Psychology, 55,* 929–948.

Farley, S. K., Sarracino, T., & Howard, P. M. (1991). Development of a treatment rating in school systems: Service through objective measurement. *American Journal of Occupational Therapy, 45*(10), 898–906.

Flaherty, J. (1999). *Coaching: Evoking excellence in others.* Boston: Butterworth-Heinemann.

Flowers, N., Mertens, S. B., & Mulhall, P. F. (1999). The impact of teaming: Five research-based outcomes. *Middle School Journal, 31*(1), 57–60.

Göncü, A. (Ed.). (1999). *Children's engagement in the world: Sociocultural perspectives*. Cambridge, UK: Cambridge University Press.

Hackman, J. R. (1987). The design of work teams. In J. Lorsch (Ed.), *Handbook of organizational behavior*. Englewood Cliffs, NJ: Prentice-Hall.

Hanft, B. E., Rush, D. D., & Shelden, M. L. (2004). *Coaching families and colleagues in early childhood*. Baltimore: Brookes.

Hoegl, M., & Gemuenden, H. G. (2001). Teamwork quality and the success of innovative projects: A theoretical concept and empirical evidence. *Organization Science, 12*, 435–449.

Individuals with Disabilities Education Act Amendments, 20 U.S.C. § 1400 *et seq.* (1997).

Joyce, B., & Showers, B. (1982). The coaching of teaching. *Educational Leadership, 40*(1), 4–8, 10.

Kinlaw, D. C. (1999). *Coaching for commitment: Interpersonal strategies for obtaining superior performance from individuals and teams*. San Francisco: Jossey-Bass.

Kohler, F. W., McCullough, K., & Buchan, K. (1995). Using peer coaching to enhance preschool teachers' development and refinement of classroom activities. *Early Intervention and Development, 6*, 215–239.

Krassowski, E., & Plante, E. (1997). IQ variability in children with SLI: Implications for use of cognitive referencing in determining SLI. *Journal of Communication Disorders, 30*, 1–9.

Larsson, M. (2000). Organising habilitation services: Team structures and family participation. *Child: Care, Health and Development, 26*, 501–514.

McWilliam, R., Ferguson, A., Harbin, G., Porter, D. M., & Vaderviere, P. (1998). The family-centeredness of individualized family services plans. *Topics in Early Childhood Special Education, 18*, 69–82.

Morgan, R. L., Gustafson, K. J., Hudson, P. J., & Salzberg, C. L. (1992). Peer coaching in a preservice special education program. *Teacher Education and Special Education, 15*, 249–258.

Munro, P., & Elliott, J. (1987). Instructional growth through peer coaching. *Journal of Staff Development, 8*(1), 25–28.

Nash, J. K. (1990). Public Law 99-457: Facilitating family participation on the multidisciplinary team. *Journal of Early Intervention, 14*, 318–326.

Notari, A. R., Cole, K. N., & Mills, P. E. (1992). Cognitive referencing: The (non)relationship between theory and application. *Topics in Early Childhood Education, 11*(4), 22–38.

Peterson, C. A., Luze, G. J., Eshbaugh, E. M., Jeon, H., & Kantz, K. R. (2007). Enhancing parent–child interaction through home visiting: Promising practice or unfulfilled promise. *Journal of Early Intervention 29*, 119–140.

Pilkington, K. O. (2006). Side by side: Transdisciplinary early intervention in natural environments. *OT Practice, 11*(6), 12–17.

Raab, M. (2005). Interest-based child participation in everyday learning activities. *CASEinPoint, 1*(2), 1–5. Available at *www.fippcase.org/caseinpoint/caseinpoint_vol1_no2.pdf*.

Rappaport, J. (1981). In praise of paradox: A social policy of empowerment over prevention. *American Journal of Community Psychology, 9*, 1–25.

Rosin, P., Whitehead, A. D., Tuchman, L. I., Jesien, G. S., Begun, A. L., & Irwin, L. (1996). *Partnerships in family-centered care: A guide to collaborative early intervention*. Baltimore: Brookes.

Rush, D., & Shelden, M. (2005). Evidence-based definition of coaching practices. *CASEin-Point, 1*(6), 1–6. Available at *www.fippcase.org/caseinpoint/caseinpoint_vol1_no6.pdf.*

Rush, D. D., Shelden, M. L., & Hanft, B. E. (2003). Coaching families and colleagues: A process for collaboration in natural settings. *Infants and Young Children, 16*, 33–47.

Sandall, S., Hemmeter, M. L., Smith, B. J., & McLean, M. E. (2005). *DEC recommended practices: A comprehensive guide for practical application in early intervention/early childhood special education.* Longmont, CA: Sopris West.

Shelden, M. L., & Rush, D. D. (2007). Characteristics of a primary coach approach to teaming in early childhood programs. *CASEinPoint, 3*(1), 1–8. Available at *www.fippcase.org/caseinpoint/caseinpoint_vol3_no1.pdf.*

Showers, B. (1985, April). Teachers coaching teachers. *Educational Leadership, 40*(7), 42–48.

Sloper, P. (2004). Facilitators and barriers for co-ordinated multi-agency services. *Child, Health, & Development, 30*, 571–580.

Sloper, P., Mukherjee, S., Beresford, B., Lightfoot, J., & Norris, P. (1999). *Real change not rhetoric: Putting research into practice in multi-agency services.* Bristol, UK: Policy Press.

Sloper, P., & Turner, S. (1992). Service needs of families of children with severe physical disability. *Child: Care, Health, and Development, 18*, 259–282.

Sparks, G. M. (1986). The effectiveness of alternative training activities in changing teaching practices. *American Educational Research Journal, 23*, 217–225.

Tarr, J. E., & Barnett, W. S. (2001). A cost analysis of Part C early intervention services in New Jersey. *Journal of Early Intervention, 24*(1), 45–54.

Trivette, C. M., & Dunst, C. J. (1998, December). *Family-centered helpgiving practices.* Paper presented at the 14th Annual Division for Early Childhood International Conference on Children with Special Needs, Chicago, IL.

Tschantz, J. M., & Vail, C. O. (2000). Effects of peer coaching on the rate of responsive teacher statements during a child-directed period in an inclusive preschool setting. *Teacher Education and Special Education, 23*, 189–201.

Vanderhoff, M. (2004). *Maximizing your role in early intervention.* Alexandria, VA: American Physical Therapy Association. Retrieved August 21, 2008, from *www.apta.org/AM/Template.cfm?Section=search&template=CM/HTMLDisplay.cfm&ContentID=8534.*

Warfield, M. E. (1995). The cost-effectiveness of home visiting versus group services in early intervention. *Journal of Early Intervention, 19*, 130–148.

Woodruff, G., & McGonigel, M. (1988). Early intervention team approaches: The transdisciplinary model. In L. J. Johnson, R. J. Gallagher, M. J. LaMontagne, J. B. Jordan, J. J. Gallagher, P. L. Huntinger, et al. (Eds.), *Early childhood special education: Birth to three* (pp. 163–181). Reston, VA: Council for Exceptional Children.

Woods, J. (2008). Providing early intervention services in natural environments. *ASHA Leader, 13*(4), 14–17, 23.

Workgroup on Principles and Practices in Natural Environments. (2007, November). *Mission and principles for providing services in natural environments.* OSEP TA Community of Practice-Part C Settings. Available at *www.nectac.org/topics/families/families.asp.*

York, J., Rainforth, B., & Giangreco, M. F. (1990). Transdisciplinary teamwork and integrated therapy: Clarifying the misconceptions. *Pediatric Physical Therapy, 2*, 73–79.

Primary-Coach Approach to Teaming Checklist

Did the practitioner . . .	✓	–	±	Comments
1. Use an approach that builds the capacity of the child's care providers to promote confidence and competence in supporting child learning within the context of natural learning environments?				
2. Use a strengths-based approach that identifies child interests and family priorities as the basis for program planning within the context of natural learning environments?				
3. Use a family-centered approach within the context of natural learning environments?				
4. Use resource-based practices to assist families in identifying, accessing, and evaluating needed and desired formal and informal resources?				
5. Assign an identified team of individuals from multiple disciplines to families in a predetermined section of the program's catchment area?				
6. Select one team member to serve as primary coach to the care provider(s)?				
7. Support the primary coach for each family in using coaching as the primary intervention strategy for building the capacity of the care providers to use everyday learning opportunities to promote child development?				
8. Support the primary coach for each family in receiving coaching from other team members?				
9. Require all team members to attend regular team meetings for the purpose of colleague-to-colleague coaching?				

(cont.)

Did the practitioner . . .	✓	–	±	Comments
10. Require other team members to visit a family/care provider only when the primary coach is present?				
11. Have a mechanism for paying team members for their time spent in team meetings, on joint visits, and coaching other colleagues?				
12. Require an identified team to support the family throughout the IFSP process (i.e., initial contact through transition)?				

CHAPTER 8

Support-Based Home Visiting

R. A. McWILLIAM

HOME VISITING IN EARLY INTERVENTION

Working with families of young children with special needs—what this book is about—when the child is younger than 3, is mostly about home visiting. Of course, other settings and events give professionals opportunities to work with families, but, as described below, the home visit is the most prevalent setting. Whereas some other chapters are concerned primarily with individualized family service plan (IFSP) development, this one, like Chapter 7 on the primary-coach approach, is concerned with week-in, week-out, ongoing interactions with families.

Seventy-two percent of children served under Part C of the Individuals with Disabilities Education Act (IDEA) are reported to be receiving services in the home (United States Department of Education, 2003). An astonishingly small literature provides evidence-based guidance about what to do on home visits to children with disabilities and their families. To confuse matters, more than one kind of home-based program for early intervention has been studied, such as those for infants born at low birthweight and prematurely, but not necessarily with disabilities (e.g., Liaw, Meisels, & Brooks-Gunn, 1995). These programs have not been based on the same principles and legislation as "Part C" home visits. Other types of home visits for infants and toddlers are British health visitors for any children (Kendrick et al., 2000), Early Head Start (Love et al., 2005), Nurses for Newborns (e.g., Korfmacher, Kitzman, & Olds, 1998), and programs for families identified as at risk of child abuse (Duggan et al., 2004). Powell (1993) discussed key dimensions to consider when viewing different home-visiting programs; these include goals, strategy for change ("home visitor–parent relationship . . . *versus* [my emphasis] dissemination of information," p. 26), host agency, content (child-related *versus* "broader ecology of family functioning," p. 26), and intensity. Notably, however, disabilities are not mentioned in Powell's review. A limited amount of research has shown home visits to be effective with families where the mother had the special needs (i.e., depression) but the child did not (e.g., Gelfand, Teti, Seiner, & Jameson, 1996). Home visitors in Part C desperately need guidance, which this chapter provides.

Family Supports and Services: A Backward-Mapping Approach

Home visiting is one of the essential methods for providing family supports. The practices that have evolved from theory, research, and experience fit into a framework tied to accountability outcomes. In a logical system of services, accountability outcomes should be tied to the actual outcomes we desire—what I have termed the moral outcomes. Indeed, it is to be hoped that outcomes for *accountability* should not drive the supports we provide families. The accountability outcomes listed in Table 8.1 are those proposed by the Early Childhood Outcomes Center and those selected by the Office of Special Education Programs (Greenwood, Walker, Bailey, & ECO Center Colleagues, 2005). The moral outcome proposed is improvement in the family's quality of life, defined as the subscales in the Beach Center's Family Quality-of-Life Measure (Park, Turnbull, & Turnbull, 2002) and McWilliam's satisfaction with routines measure (McWilliam, 2005b).

TABLE 8.1. Backward-Mapping Framework for Family Supports and Services

Infrastructure	Practices ←	Content ←	Moral outcome ↔	Accountability outcomes
• Primary service provider (transdisciplinary) • Blended-model service coordinator • Support for primary service provider (other services) • Well-trained personnel • Policies to support natural environments	• Ecomap • Routines-Based Interview • Support-based home visits, including emotional support: • Positiveness • Responsiveness • Orientation to the whole family • Friendliness • Sensitivity	• Family's ecology • Information to family about: • Child development • Resources, including services • Child's disability or condition • What to do with child • Rights	• Other • *Family quality of life* • Family interaction (T) • General resources (T) • Health and safety (T) • Parenting (T) • Satisfaction with routines (M)	• Understand their child's strengths, abilities, and special needs (ECO) • Know their rights and advocate effectively for their children (ECO and OSEP) • Help their child develop and learn (ECO and OSEP) • Have support systems (ECO) • Access desired services, programs, and activities in their community (ECO)

Note. T: Park et al. (2003); M: McWilliam (2005a, 2005b); ECO: Greenwood et al. (2005); OSEP: Office of Special Education Programs, U.S. Department of Education.

If the primary moral outcome is the improvement of families' quality of life, what do we need to attend to on home visits? Two content areas are the family's ecology and informational support. Understanding the family's ecology is essential for (1) letting the family know that home visits are about the whole family, not just the "client" child; and (2) knowing what informal and formal supports are available to the family (Harbin, 2005). Informational support is one of the foundations of support-based home visits (McWilliam & Scott, 2001). Note that one of the types of information provided to families is what to do with the child. This is a highly significant content area, because it is has been the focus of home visits over the years. It is proposed in this model that speech–language services, special instruction, occupational therapy, and physical therapy in the context of home visits in early intervention are, in fact, the provision of informational support to families.

The significance of this proposition is that the clinic-based approach, emphasizing the hands-on work by the professional, consists of a minimal stress on providing information to regular caregivers. In that model, professionals work with the child, sometimes in the belief that they are modeling for the family. Sometimes, such as when the family is not even in the room, not even modeling is the purpose: The purpose is direct treatment. Professionals might say, "Try this during the week." Note that what families are asked to try does not necessarily fit into their routines, because they were demonstrated in the artificial context of the home visit. In fact, it is little better than a strategy shown in a clinic, which is why we have dubbed this a "clinic-based model dumped on the living room floor" (McWilliam, 1998).

If home visits should include providing information to the family, as shown in Table 8.1, what should be the practices or processes to address that content? In this model, those practices are as follows:

1. The ecomap for understanding families' routines.
2. The Routines-Based Interview (McWilliam, 1992, 2005a) (1) to establish a positive relationship with the family, (2) to assess the family's functional needs; and (3) to help the family decide on their priorities for intervention.
3. Emotional support to encourage families.
4. Informational support to increase families' knowledge and skills.

These practices can be implemented in a number of infrastructure arrangements, but what contexts are best for such implementation?

1. A primary service provider model sets the stage for the family to receive a comprehensive set of interventions, rather than the scattershot approach characteristic of a multidisciplinary approach (Hanft, Rush, & Shelden, 2004).
2. A service coordinator model that allows the primary (or a primary) ser-

vice provider to function also as the service coordinator (Bruder & Dunst, 2006).

3. A team of professionals with disparate skill and knowledge sets who, together, back up the primary service provider.

4. A cadre of professionals who are very knowledgeable about child development (normal and abnormal), family functioning, and consultation (including adult education).

5. A method to pay for travel time so services are provided in natural environments.

This logical framework ties together the necessary elements of a system of early intervention. It is preferable to the cobbled-together approach that can be the result of politics, history, payment structures, and misinformation about how children learn and how interventions work.

The FACINATE Context

In providing early intervention, five key elements are linked to form a model called FACINATE: FAmily-Centered Interventions in NATural Environments. The key elements of this model—(1) understanding the family ecology, (2) routines-based assessment, (3) the primary service provider, (4) support-based home visits, and (5) collaborative child care consultation—are shown in Figure 8.1. Most of these key elements have been mentioned already. Collaborative child care consultation is beyond the scope of this chapter, but it should be noted that it consists of inte-

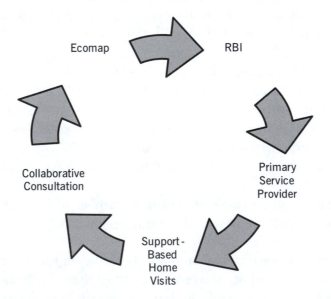

FIGURE 8.1. Key elements of the FACINATE model of early intervention.

grating the consultation into the classroom routines. Children are not pulled out for instruction or therapy. This is consistent with the routines-based approach in home visits.

THE NEED FOR GUIDELINES FOR HOME VISITORS

Because of the relative lack of attention to home-visiting practices in the literature and equally because of my experience in assisting states and programs in implementing support-based home visits, this chapter addresses the need for a set of written guidelines. The guidelines need to address four persistent problems in early intervention. First, the pernicious slide toward overspecialization has advanced a notion that every need requires a service. This can be seen when an early intervention family has a host of specialists making frequent visits. Second, an erroneous belief that more is better, when it comes to the number and intensity of services, has led to the pile-on effect just described. The problem as applied to intensity of any one service is ludicrously seen when a child makes little progress in an area being addressed by a particular service (e.g., a therapy), so the team decides to increase the intensity—as though that were the answer. Third, the failure of professionals to take responsibility for families' difficulty in selecting outcomes has led to pathetically weak IFSPs, where target behaviors are poorly described, criteria for attainment are either absent or nonsensical, and strategies do not match outcomes (Jung & McWilliam, 2005). Fourth, the clinic- or classroom-based model of intervention, dumped on the living room floor, has robbed families of the information they need to provide children with context-relevant developmental help. (See Appendix 8.1, Support-Based Home-Visiting Checklist, at the end of this chapter.)

The Misplaced Clinic-Based Approach

The misplaced clinic-based approach has typically been focused on the toy bag, the ubiquitous crutch of the traditional home visitor. The toy bag implies the family's materials are not good enough, contains toys that are then removed at the end of the home visit, and sets the agenda, in that traditional home visitors went through the toys, one by one. Giving up the toy bag is one of the hardest aspects of this model, so strong is the addiction.

Another characteristic of dumping the clinic-based approach on the living room floor, as it were, is that the home visitor "works with" the child. This implies that the child learns from the visitor, which is misleading for the family. Working with the child directly also leads to complaints about the family's lack of "involvement" during the home visit. Not surprisingly, families who see the professional working with their child might think that this is a good opportunity to catch up on laundry or the soap operas, prompting the professional to lament lack of family involvement. In general, in the clinic-based approach, the family's primary role is to observe.

There are four problems with this approach:

1. It suggests that child change occurs as a result of home visits, rather than as a result of all the family–child interactions and other adult–child interactions that occur between visits.
2. It oversimplifies the needs that should be addressed in home visits, as though they were simply to provide developmental interventions to the child, which leads to the next problem.
3. It promotes the *got a need, get a service* mentality, requiring a specialist for every need.
4. It falls victim to the *model and pray* notion of how home visits work; that is, that the home visitor models and then prays the family was attending and imitates later.

These problems in early intervention can be addressed with a home visiting framework based on five key principles.

The Five Key Principles You Need to Understand about This Model

1. *It's the family that influences the child, and we can influence the family.* Families have greater influence over children than do home visitors who might see the child for 1 hour a week (McWilliam, 2003).
2. *Children learn throughout the day.* Young children do not learn in clumps of instruction or therapy that requires the processing of multiple rapid-fire inputs (i.e., massed trials; Grisham-Brown, Schuster, Hemmeter, & Collins, 2000).
3. *Early intervention is not about providing weekly lessons.* In addition to the fact that young children learn through distributed trials, they have difficulty transferring from decontextualized settings to regular routines.
4. *All the intervention for the child occurs between visits.* Because of the first three principles above, the function of the home visit needs to shift from direct intervention with the child to support of the caregivers.
5. *It's maximal intervention the child needs, not maximal services.* If the first four principles above are followed, the child's many learning opportunities are maximized and optimized. Regular caregivers' interventions with children are not affected by having more professionals providing more services.

The difference between intervention and service is important for understanding the role of home visits. Intervention is what the child receives, and service is what the caregivers (families and child care providers) receive.

These five principles have been influenced by Bruder's (e.g., 2000) clarifications of family-centered early intervention; Campbell's (1987) description of the integrated-programming team; Dunst's and Trivette's (1988) elaborations of social support, (and with Bruder) learning opportunities, and service coordination (e.g., Dunst, 2001; Dunst & Trivette, 1988; Dunst, Hamby, Trivette, Raab, & Bruder, 2002); McBride's and Peterson's (1997) research on home-visiting practices; Roberts's Rule's, and Innocenti's (e.g., 1998) work on family–professional partnerships; Edelman's (2001) articulation of team models for different disciplines to work together; Hanft et al.'s (2004) primary-coach model; and Woods's and Wetherby's (e.g., 2003) work on embedding intervention in daily routines. The model draws on this body of literature to set the stage for support-based home visits.

Asssumptions

For successful, support-based home visits to occur, four assumptions must be met.

Assumption 1

The first assumption is that we have introduced the FACINATE model early on, so families are not surprised by subsequent approaches we take. When we introduce the model we emphasize that

- We maximize interventions to children.
- More interventions do not come from more services.
- All the intervention occurs between visits.
- The job of professionals is to support regular caregivers. This support is articulated in the following promise we can make to families:

We will inform you.
We will teach you how to teach and do other things with your child.
We will tell you about your child's disability.
We will tell you about resources.
We will teach you about child development.
We will give you access to materials you need.
We will get equipment, including assistive technology, you need to help your child's development.
We will make sure you have access to financial resources that you're entitled to.
We will support you, emotionally.
We will be positive with and about you.
We will be responsive to you.
We will pay attention to your whole family, especially the primary caregiver.
We will be friendly to you.
We will be sensitive to you.

Assumption 2

The second assumption is that we know who is in the family and who important members of the informal, formal, and intermediate support networks are. This is best accomplished by conducting an ecomap.

Assumption 3

The third assumption is that we have a list of functional outcomes or goals, truly decided upon by the family (as opposed to a list decided upon by professionals and approved by the family). Functional outcomes or goals would be based on in-depth assessment of family routines and would be placed into the order of importance to the family.

Assumption 4

The fourth assumption is that the home visitor supports the family with all outcomes or goals, not just some outcomes or goals specific to one discipline. The primary service provider model (e.g., primary coach, transdisciplinary) allows for this type of support, compared to the multidisciplinary or interdisciplinary models, in which home visitors address only those outcomes or goals within their discipline.

The model presented here can be used if one or two of these assumptions are violated, but it is greatly enhanced if they all are followed. Now the early interventionist is ready to provide support-based home visits.

Three Forms of Support

The alternative to the clinic-based model being dumped on the living room floor is support-based home visits (McWilliam, 2000, 2002; McWilliam & Scott, 2001; McWilliam, Snyder, Harbin, Porter, & Munn, 2000). This approach to home visiting revolves around three types of support not unlike Guralnick's (1998, 2001) developmental-systems model for early intervention.

Emotional Support

In a qualitative study of family-centered service delivery in early intervention for children up to age 5 (McWilliam, Tocci, & Harbin, 1998), five key characteristics of emotionally supportive professionals were discovered:

1. *Positiveness.* Being positive to and about both children and family members.
2. *Responsiveness.* Offering to do something when the family expresses a concern and following through in general.

3. *Orientation to the whole family.* Acknowledging family members, especially the primary caregiver, and their needs.
4. *Friendliness.* Treating families like neighbors not clients.
5. *Sensitivity.* Walking in the family's shoes, including not giving them homework they do not want or to be done at inconvenient times.

Other dimensions of emotional support such as empathy and encouragement are important also.

Material Support

Providing material support involves ensuring the family has access to (1) materials and equipment, and (2) financial resources. Materials include necessities such as shelter, clothing, transport, food, and diapers. Being in the home gives the professional the opportunity to see whether these are adequate. If not, they should be the first priority. The home visitor should ensure, directly or indirectly, that the family has access to these materials. Direct support would entail working with agencies and the family. Indirect support would entail passing off this responsibility to another professional, such as a service coordinator, if the home visitor did not have that role.

Equipment consists of the structural supports a child needs to be engaged and independent and have social relationships during routines, such as adaptive seating and communication boards. It can also consist of positioning devices and exercise aids such as wedges, bolsters, therapy balls, corner chairs, and prone standers. Home visitors should help families maintain as normal a home as the family wants, however, by limiting the "abnormal" equipment to what is necessary for successful functioning. Crowding a small living room with exercise equipment for which there is scant evidence of effectiveness might not be in the family's best interest. Whenever possible, home visitors should help families use everyday materials.

Informational Support

When families are asked what more they want from their early intervention providers, they often say information (Sontag & Schacht, 1993). They want information about four things home visitors should be prepared to provide.

1. *Child development.* Families want to know what other children their child's age can do or what comes next, developmentally. Home visitors should be trained to have this information.
2. *Child's disability.* Families want to know about their child's disability or condition. They also sometimes know more about it than does the home visitor. Again, home visitors should know about the most common disabilities or be able to get information about those disabilities they do not know about.

3. *Services and resources.* Families want to know where they can get help and where learning opportunities might exist. The concern about services becomes quite focused at transitions, as the family is preparing to change service providers. Home visitors should know about the resources in their community or where to obtain that information.

4. *What to do with the child.* This is the main part of informational support that early interventionists have traditionally provided, and it will continue to be a very important part. Because the provision of pediatric therapy (occupational therapy [OT], physical therapy [PT], and speech–language pathology [SLP]) and early childhood special education is giving families knowledge and skills (i.e., information) about what they can do in regular routines to help their child, therapy and education in early intervention is actually a form of providing informational support. Framing them as support might help therapists and teachers understand the basic consultative role of their jobs.

Professionals should therefore make home visits with the goals of providing emotional, material, and informational support.

A FRAMEWORK FOR HOME VISITS

A mechanism for helping home visitors focus on support is the Vanderbilt Home Visit Script (VHVS; McWilliam, 2004), shown in Appendix 8.2 at the end of this chapter. It provides home visitors with the agenda they miss when they do not take a toy bag into the home, because the toys in toy-bag-based home visits are the agenda.

Appropriate Use of the Script

The following passage shows the skepticism some leaders in the field have had about the impact of home visits on caregivers' intervening with children intensely enough, without turning them into therapists and teachers:

> Clearly every interaction an infant experiences throughout the day has the potential to influence development. To what extent can weekly home visits and therapy sessions in which professionals interact directly with the child be expected to produce significant benefit? Hanft and Feinberg [1997] have argued that this question cannot be answered without considering child needs and the desires of individual families. Perhaps if the visits are designed to help caregivers structure and support children's usual interactions, more benefit can be expected. However, such approaches, if done inappropriately, may place demands on families to become teachers and therapists and may lead to unintended negative outcomes. Furthermore, the efficacy of home visiting alone as a means of altering developmental pathways for children with disabilities has not been demonstrated. Structuring interventions to impact children's

usual and day-long interactions will require interventionists to know the contexts in which children spend time; the usual activities, and events in those contexts; the behaviors of adults in those contexts; and children's interest in and reaction to those events, routines, and activities. They will also need to be able to work effectively with families to encourage the application of intervention activities across daily routines. (Bailey, Aytch, Odom, Symons, & Wolery, 1999, pp. 14-15)

The VHVS is designed to help early interventionists work with families like this.

Content

The script comes with directions, guidelines for follow-up questions, and seven lead questions. It is written for home visits by primary service providers (i.e., professionals following a transdisciplinary service delivery model) but it can be adapted for use by multidisciplinary providers. At any time during the interview following this protocol, the early interventionist should provide support to the family, including information.

Follow-Up Prompts for All Script Questions

To ensure home visitors provide emotional support, they are prompted to attend to "the four E's":

- Ears (listen)
- Elicit (ask)
- Empathize
- Encourage

Furthermore, at any time during the interview, they should be prepared to ask the following three questions:

1. Do you need any information to help with this?
2. Should we try to solve this?
3. Would you like me to show you?

The four E's and the offers to provide information, solutions, and demonstration set the tone for the home visit based on emotional and informational support, including information about material support.

Lead Questions

In the VHVS, seven lead questions constitute the structure, but one of these—the third question—is about each outcome. So, in a sense, each outcome carries a lead question, giving us 12 or more (assuming 6–10 functional, family-centered out-comes) potential lead questions. Many home visits will not last long enough to address all the questions.

1. *How have things been going?* This ordinary first question could be the last lead question asked in a single visit, if it generates a lengthy, involved discussion, or it could be simply answered with "OK," "Good," or whatever. It gives the family an opportunity to set the agenda. Although it is a familiar first question, therefore, the answer should sometimes be taken seriously, if the family elaborates on the answer. *Remember, at any point in discussing the answer to this or any other question, the home visitor can offer information, joint problem solving, and demonstration of techniques.*

2. *Do you have anything new you want to ask me about?* The idea is not nec-essarily to set the home visitor up as the expert, so it can be worded, "Do you have anything new you want to talk about?" As with all questions, this one should be paraphrased to suit the people involved. It gives the family a more specific oppor-tunity than the first question to think about new issues, skills, problems, and so on.

3. *Outcomes in priority order.* The home visit will go much more smoothly if the goals are functional, preferably based on needs in the family's routines. They are asked in the order of importance the family chose in the development of the IFSP. The question would often be "How have things been going with sitting inde-pendently when Raúl is playing with Alejandra?" or whatever the first priority is. It might work just to ask, "How have things been going with sitting?" But, as soon as discussion ensues, it is important to ask about sitting during specific rou-tines, such as, "*When* have you noticed he falls over?" Functionality almost always hinges on the child's functioning in specific situations, because children respond to external stimuli. For example, Raúl's sitting independently in the living room might be hard for him because he keeps turning his head to look at the family dog running around. On the other hand, at night, when he's sitting in his crib, he might do better with the different surface (mattress versus floor) and fewer distrac-tions. Therefore, potential solutions (i.e., interventions) will vary by routine. If the Routines-Based Interview (RBI; McWilliam, 1992, 2005a) was used, there should be 6–10 goals, so it is very likely not all the goals will be covered in a single home visit. From time to time, the home visitor might suggest starting with goals further down the priority list, to make sure none are ignored for weeks on end.

4. *Is there a time of day that's not going well for you?* If, miraculously, the discussion of goals does not consume the whole home visit, this question can be helpful for families. It is highly relevant if we believe that helping families increase their satisfaction with routines is a purpose of early intervention.

5. *How is [family member] doing?* Because family-centered practices include an orientation to the whole family (McWilliam et al., 1998), it is important to ask about family members other than the target child. Very often, this family member

should be the very person being visited, such as the mother. The question is also pertinent because the child lives in the context of a family.

6. *Have you had any appointments in the past week? Any coming up?* Answering these questions can help organize the information the family received at an appointment or organize questions to ask professionals at an upcoming appointment. Keeping up with the information and paperwork related to assessments and check-ups can be challenging for many families of all kinds of backgrounds. It is good not to make assumptions either that the family has all this information under control or that they do not.

7. *Do you have enough or too much to do with [your child]?* Although we might have a sense of whether the number of suggestions is more or less than the family wants, it is good to check in with them. If nothing else, asking the question demonstrates the home visitor's sensitivity to the family's desire for amount of advice.

It is unlikely the home visitor will reach all these steps on any home visit, which illustrates a couple of important points. First, there is a lot to do on a support-based home visit, especially considering that the RBI even for children with mild delays will have 6–10 functional outcomes. Because these home visits are very busy, it is difficult to imagine how a reasonable level of support could be achieved without weekly visits. A more dispersed schedule (e.g., twice a month) is likely to suit more narrowly focused visits with fewer outcomes. Second, the VHVS is a reasonable substitute for other agendas, such as toy bags. On first inspection, one might think that seven questions will leave the home visitor and family stranded with nothing to do, but in fact it is a very full agenda. Should home visits be scripted? Note that the agenda consists of prompt questions to ask the family about their priorities. The script encompasses only the lead questions; all the meat of the conversation is in the responses and follow-ups.

What Will Home Visits Look Like?

Home visitors might be afraid home visits will no longer involve interaction between them and the child. It is true that the focus is no longer on that interaction. In some models, the focus is on the interaction between the adult family member (we'll refer to that person as the parent) and the child. Here, that is somewhat of a focus, but the real focus is on the interaction between the home visitor and the parent—on the topic of the interaction of the parent and the child. That is, the home visitor uses appropriate consultative and adult-education strategies to help the parent teach and in other ways intervene with the child.

Home visitors in this model will spend much time talking to the family, but most of the time they will still have their hands on the child. For many home visitors, hands-on contact with children is very important. The three reasons for "handling" the child are (1) to demonstrate intervention strategies; (2) to assess what the child can do or what might work, before making the suggestion to the family; and (3) to show the parent that the home visitor loves the child. Long after early intervention has ended, families might not remember their home visitor's name and certainly not his or her degrees, but they will remember that he or she loved their child.

The Eight Steps of Modeling: Avoiding the Model-and-Pray Approach

One of the reasons for handling the child is demonstration. In the past, some home visitors who "worked with" the child on home visits would claim they were directly teaching or providing therapy to the child. Those with more understanding about how children learn and how services work would claim they were demonstrating for the parent. Too often, however, the demonstration was clearly not working. This could be seen either by nonengaged parents, who might be talking on the telephone, watching television, or doing laundry during the visit; or, on subsequent visits, parents' revealing they had not imitated what the home visitor had modeled. Such home visitors use the model-and-pray approach. That is, they model and pray that the parent was observing and will spontaneously imitate the model during the week. The antidote to the model-and-pray approach is the eight steps of modeling:

1. Talk to the parent about your suggestion.
2. If the parent appears not to understand, ask if he or she would like to be shown.
3. Tell the parent what you're going to do.
4. Do it.
5. Tell the parent what you did and point out the consequence.
6. Ask the parent if he or she would like to try it.
7. If the answer is "yes," watch the parent trying it; if the answer is "no," leave it alone.
8. If yes, praise the parent and give a limited amount of corrective feedback.

Here is how the eight steps would work when demonstrating to a parent a backward-chaining, full physical prompt to teach the child independent eating with a spoon.

1. "Have you considered standing behind him and help him at the elbow, letting go at the last minute, so he finishes the act of eating with a spoon by himself?" (Talk to the parent about your suggestion.)
2. "I can tell I haven't explained this very well. Would you like me to show you what I'm talking about?" (If the parent appears not to understand, ask if he or she would like to be shown.)

3. "I'm going to stand behind him while he's in the high chair. I'm going to say, 'Time to eat' and then I'm going to hold his elbow, lightly, to guide him to scoop and bring his food to his mouth. When the spoon gets close to his mouth, I'm going to let go of his elbow, so he'll put the spoon in his mouth by himself." (Tell the parent what you're going to do.)
4. "See what I'm doing." (Do it.)
5. "Did you see how I stood behind him? I said, 'Time to eat' and then I held his elbow, lightly, to guide him to scoop and bring his food to his mouth. When the spoon got close to his mouth, I let go of his elbow, so he put the spoon in his mouth by himself." (Tell the parent what you did and point out the consequence.)
6. "Would you like to try teaching him like that?" (Ask the parent if he or she would like to try it.)
7. "You go ahead and do it and I'll watch you and coach you as necessary!" (If the answer is "yes," watch the parent trying it.)
"If you try it and have any questions next time I'm here, let me know." (If the answer is "no," leave it alone.)
8. "That was excellent! You guided him gently, so he scooped well and brought the spoon to his mouth. Next time, remember to let go of his elbow, so he can do the last part himself." (If yes, praise the parent and give a limited amount of corrective feedback.)

Transdisciplinary Service Delivery

The transdisciplinary approach to service delivery, also known as the primary service provider model or the primary-coach model, is described by Shelden and Rush (Chapter 7, this volume). Because this approach (1) integrates strategies from different disciplines, (2) enhances the relationship of a primary service provider (PSP) and the family, and (3) lowers the burden of participating in professional services for the family (thereby giving them more time to do other things), it is supported in the VHVS. It is consistent with the five key principles listed earlier in this chapter.

Implications for Specialists' Roles

Unfortunately, some therapists fear this model makes them irrelevant. Nothing could be further from the truth. This model requires them to be critical team members and to work with the family to devise appropriate programs of intervention. The difference is that this model focuses on natural caregivers carrying out the interventions throughout the day, thus maximizing the child's learning opportunities. The therapist does not need to be around as often, when the interventions are in the hands of the caregivers. The job of the primary service provider (i.e., the regular home visitor) is to support the family in carrying out those interventions and to summon the assistance of the therapist when needed. Note that a therapist can be a PSP and summon the assistance of the generalist when needed. Therefore, therapists are needed just as much as ever, but they need to be used differently from the traditional approach of every professional on the team seeing the family frequently.

In addition to the role release required of therapists with this model, therapists need to develop consultative skills as part of "direct therapy." Professional organizations' descriptions of therapy with very young children recognize that "parent education" is a key part of direct therapy, and that is the part that is so critical to the PSP model.

FUNCTIONAL CHILD DOMAINS

As home visitors work with families, they seek to determine needs (see R. A. McWilliam, Chapter 2, this volume) and they provide various types of support. What developmental, behavioral, and ecological framework do they use for assessing and suggesting interventions? Traditionally, they have used domains found in norm-referenced tests and in curricula, such as cognitive, communication, motor, social, and adaptive. A more functional set of domains has been proposed as engagement, independence, and social relationships (see R. A. McWilliam, Chapter 2, this volume).

Engagement

Engagement is the amount of time a child spends interacting competently with the environment (McWilliam & Bailey, 1992). It is closely related to the concept of participation, which the World Health Organization (2007) has emphasized as a criterion for functioning. That is, a person with an impairment is less functionally "handicapped" the more he or she can participate in home, school, work, or community routines. For very young children, the observable and measurable equivalent of participation in routines is engagement.

Historically, engagement was thought of as simply on task or off task (e.g., Risley & Cataldo, 1973). More recent research in early intervention/early childhood special education (ECSE), however, has considered engagement at different levels of sophistication. High-level engagement consists of mastery behaviors, constructive play, and encoded social interactions (e.g., conventionalized language and rule following; de Kruif & McWilliam, 1999; Dunst & McWilliam, 1988). Middle-level engagement consists of neither sophisticated nor low-level participation in routines, but differentiated behavior and focused attention. Low-level engagement consists of undifferentiated behavior (i.e., repetitive actions) and casual attention. Nonengagement can be active, involving crying or being aggressive, or passive, involving needlessly waiting, staring into space, or wandering aimlessly. On home visits, professionals work with families to determine the amount and sophistication of a child's engagement in each routine and to improve it. The assessment process is best done through a semistructured interview to cover the many ways in which a child could be engaged and to allow the family and the home visitor to ensure they understand each other's concepts of engagement.

Independence

The second new "domain" is independence, which is often concomitant with engagement. That is, children who are more independent in a routine tend to be more engaged in it. To make this functional on home visits, professionals are interested in independence only in everyday routines, not in tests or other decontextualized events. They need to consider cultural norms and individual–family preferences about the extent of a child's independence. Some families believe the role of parents is to do things for children, so they might be less interested in this domain than are other families.

Social Relationships

The third new domain is social relationships, which is the ability to interact successfully with people in the environment. It thus consists of communication and getting along with others. Again, it is not mutually exclusive of engagement. Childen who are competently involved in social relationships will be more engaged than are those who do not have successful social relationships.

If home visitors keep their focus on engagement, independence, and social relationships, they are likely to deal with meaningful functioning and to avoid the pile-on of different services at a high intensity.

TEACHING PARENTS TO TEACH THEIR CHILDREN

The consultative approach is a good and correct one in home visiting, but there are times when parents want to learn specific strategies. The rationale for "training" parents, some key child-instruction strategies, and the use of performance feedback for parent training are discussed.

Rationale and Apology

When families want to know what to do with their children—when that is the type of informational support they are seeking, the home visitor should be able to teach them what to do. Sometimes, other team members are needed to arrive at specific strategies. Parents decide what it is they want their children to do: They are generally able to say what functional behaviors they want to see in their children (e.g., nursing, playing back-and-forth games, walking, communicating). But they might not know how to teach these skills to children. One reason might be because the child has difficulty learning or performing the skill. Unlike typically developing children, whose learning, by and large, matches the input from the parents, children with disabilities or difficult temperaments might not be as easy to teach. Even among typically developing children, ease of teaching varies considerably.

A second reason parents might want specific training in what to do with their child is their own difficulty in understanding less structured suggestions. If a home visitor makes a suggestion about what a parent can do to help address a child-level need the parent has expressed, the parent might not really understand how to incorporate that suggestion into everyday life. For example, the parent might say she wants her child to be able to scoop oatmeal with a spoon and feed herself with little spilling. The home visitor might tell the parent about providing full physical assistance in the form of hand over hand, then fading the assistance by moving the prompt up the arm. Let us assume the home visitor makes this suggestion well, offering to demonstrate and to give feedback as the parent tries it. If the parent indicates, on a subsequent home visit, that she did not really understand the timing involved in this prompt-fading procedure, and that she is frustrated because she feels she is not teaching her child effectively, the home visitor can offer to teach her the prompt-fading procedure more systematically. This concept of moving from suggestion only to parent training is discussed in the section "Three Tiers for Response to Intervention" section later in this chapter.

A third reason to incorporate actual parent training might be because a desired child behavior is of very high priority for a family. They might be very bothered by the child's inability to perform a skill, by the child's behavior, or by external pressure for the child to be able to perform a skill. For example, a grandparent of the child's might be putting the pressure on the parents, or the child care program is withholding promotion to the next age group until the child learns some particular skills. When the family has placed a child skill as a high priority, they might want more systematic help than simply suggestions. Therefore, if the child has great difficulty in learning a skill, the parent has difficulty in learning an intervention, or the skill has assumed a mighty importance, systematic instruction of parents might be warranted.

Key Child-Instruction Strategies

What are important intervention skills, cutting across routines and developmental domains, for parents to learn?

The first is incidental teaching as described in the 1970s by Hart and Risley (1974; 1975). Although originally designed for teaching language, this strategy can be applied across routines and domains. It involves setting up the environment, if necessary; observing the child's engagement (i.e., what the child is interested in); and eliciting a specific behavior, longer engagement, or more sophisticated engagement (McWilliam, Wolery, & Odom, 2001). The home visitor first teaches the parent to observe the child's engagement by noting what the child is looking at, what objects he or she is handling, or who the child seems interested in. Families thereby learn to answer the question, at any time, "What is my child interested in right now?" The home visitor then teaches parents how to elicit longer interaction with the object (human or material) of the child's interest, more sophisticated interaction, or a specific interaction. Longer interactions involve helping the child see the object or person in a continuously reinforcing light—keeping it interesting. More sophisticated interactions can include adding in language, more differentiated behavior (i.e., doing different things with the person or object), or problem solving with the person or object (such as by making the interaction challenging enough that the child has to figure out how to continue the interaction, but not so challenging that the child gives up).

The second general strategy can be the systematic application of reinforcement principles (Premack, 1959). Parents can be taught to apply reinforcers, to withhold them, to schedule them, to deliver them at different levels of intensity, and so on (Horner, Dunlap, & Koegel, 1988). Families can be taught the general principles of antecedents, behaviors, and consequences (ABC), so they can make their teaching most effective. They learn to pay attention to setting events and discriminative stimuli, to focus on the specific behavior they are teaching the child to engage in, and to ensure they are providing reinforcers for skills they want to see more of and withholding sometimes inadvertently reinforcers for actions they want to see less of.

The third strategy might be time delay, which is not simply waiting for a response. It is the planned timing between the task direction (e.g., "Time to eat") and the controlling prompt (e.g., taking the child by the hand and leading him or her to the table) (Wolery, Anthony, Caldwell, Snyder, & Morgante, 2002). The home visitor might teach the parent to have no time between the task direction and the controlling prompt, so "errorless learning" occurs; the child doesn't have a chance to make a mistake. Gradually, the delay between the task direction and the prompt is increased, as the child becomes more competent at the skill.

All three of these strategies, incidental teaching, reinforcement, and time delay, are *teaching* strategies that can be used across routines and domains. Home visitors vary greatly in their knowledge of specific teaching strategies and, perhaps more important, in their ability to educate adults on how to use them.

Three Tiers for Response to Intervention

Home visits should be tailored to the family's interests, including their interest in learning specific strategies or techniques to use with the child. One approach to this might be to adopt the three-tiered approach common in school psychology (Kratochwill, Albers, & Shernoff, 2004) and the response-to-intervention framework in school-age special education (Danielson, Doolittle, & Bradley, 2007;

Gresham, 2007). This approach is commonly depicted as a triangle with universal and preventive services in the bottom section. If those services are not effective, a set of intervention services is offered—the middle section of the triangle, showing that this is for a smaller number of children or families. Finally, Tier 3 is the top of the triangle, where intensive, highly individualized services are offered. A model for parent education, following the three-tier model, in the context of preschool (children ages 3–5 years) services, has been proposed (McIntyre & Phaneuf, 2007); it consists of (1) "family-focused early childhood education; self-administered parent education materials"; (2) "group-based parent education"; and (3) "1:1 support" (p. 218). A home-based model for families of infants and toddlers receiving Part C services could also use the three-tier approach (see Figure 8.2).

Regular home visits, as described in this chapter, can be offered to all families in Part C. This is the least intrusive level or tier. As the home visitor makes sug-

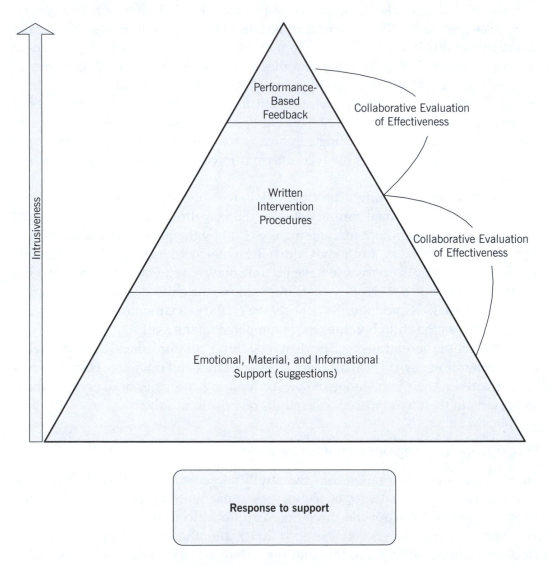

FIGURE 8.2. Response to support.

gestions, as part of providing support, together he or she and the parent ask, "Is this level of support working for the family in terms of parent implementation or of child performance for each outcome?" If the answer is "yes," Tier 1 continues for each outcome. If, for one or more outcomes, the answer is "no," the home visitor provides the family with written or symbolic intervention procedures. Symbolic procedures might be visual schedules or task analyses, which might be helpful for people who do not read the home visitor's language. If this level is mutually determined not to be effective, the family is offered a more intensive and intrusive form of support: performance-based feedback.

Training Parents through Performance Feedback

Parent education is a controversial issue in early intervention. Some experts believe that it is a narrow and paternalistic role to take with families (Dunst, 1999). Other experts believe that it is the essence of supporting families who want to know what to do with their child (Kaiser et al., 1999; Mahoney et al., 1999). It is possible that the response-to-support model proposed in this chapter allows for both perspectives, beginning with the proactive, unintrusive approach and moving to more of an educational, intrusive approach, as the families request it.

Performance feedback is the systematic delivery of information to a learner about his or her actions. When working with parents in home visits, three dimensions of feedback need to be considered. First, checklists can be developed to lay out the steps of the intervention with the child, to provide a platform for giving feedback, and to monitor the parent's performance to know whether the intervention is being carried out as planned. Second, the home visitor uses the checklists to observe the parent showing how he or she intervenes with the child during the week when the home visitor is not there. The home visitor then provides specific feedback, based on the checklists. Third, the family uses the checklists for self-monitoring, which will be successful for some families and not for others. Using checklists, observing, giving feedback, and supporting self-monitoring can all be done in a family-centered manner, if the family wants this level of training.

An example of the use of feedback would be if the family decided they wanted to know how to wash their child's hair in a way that didn't cause the child to scream and kick. The home visitor had tried various suggestions (Tier 1) and had given the family some written guidelines (Tier 2), but the family felt they were not doing it right, because the child was still screaming and kicking. The home visitor then observed bathing and talked to the parents at length about how the bath-time routine worked. This is essentially a functional behavior assessment, producing the finding that the child screamed and kicked to avoid getting his hair wet. This is known as an escape function for the behavior. The home visitor then proposed a bath-time procedure with very detailed steps. The procedure involved setting a fun bath-time atmosphere and then shaping the child's tolerance of wet hair. At first, the parent was instructed to place a wet hand on the back of the child's hair and also instructed on how to document what the parent did and what the child did. Data collection is very important in parent training through perfor-mance feedback. The home visitor taught the parent how the child had to tolerate having a wet hand on his head for three consecutive bath times before the parent moved on to the next level, which was to use a hand to drip water on to the back of the child's head. The home visitor explained that, over several weeks, as the child became more tolerant of these little steps toward getting hair wet, the amount of water increased. The feedback the home visitor provided was based on both the data the parent collected during the week and on the home visitor's observation of the parent's teaching the child. Parent training through feedback is an intensive level of support to families, so it is reserved for situations where easier and less invasive strategies have not worked.

CHALLENGING SITUATIONS IN HOME VISITING

Some families provide especially challenging situations for home visitors. These can be the most interesting and simpáticas families. Four types are discussed.

Families Who Don't Follow Through with Interventions

When this happens, it is the home visitor's responsibility. Blaming the family is not only countertheoretical but futile. The three most common reasons for families not to follow through are (1) the outcome has little meaning, (2) the suggested interven-tion does not fit into the family's routine or frame of reference, and (3) they have competing priorities. This indeed is the order in which to address the lack of fol-low through. First, interventionists should ensure the outcomes are derived from needs the family has identified in a routines-based assessment. Next, intervention-ists should try different suggestions for the family. Finally, interventionists should rethink how they are supporting the family. If the family has competing priorities, interventionists can support the families with those priorities, if they are appropri-ate; this is, after all, a family-centered service. Interventionists should know that their ethical obligation is to ensure the family has information. For example, if the family is not working on skills they have themselves identified as important, inter-ventionists can gently point out the likely consequences. It is extremely important to be ethical about providing this information, because families' failure to "follow through" is not usually neglect or a life-or-death situation.

Families Who Have Been Coerced into Services

Some families receive home visits because they were referred to early intervention by the public social services agency. These families might believe there is nothing wrong with their child, they might not trust the early intervention professionals, and they might resent having to receive these services. Even when they are told the program is voluntary, they might (perhaps accurately) perceive participation to be obligatory if they are to keep their children. The four keys to making successful home visits with such families are as follows.

1. Conduct a Routines-Based Interview, because this focuses on what the parent wants the child and other family members to do to make routines more satisfactory. It does not assume a disability.
2. Work to ensure the family understands that the home visitor is there to make the life of the family more pleasant, as defined by the family.
3. Be prepared to spend much energy on fostering a personal relationship with the parent and on helping the family secure resources such as governmental support.
4. Offer the family almost unconditionally positive feedback about what they do with their children. This builds the relationship to the point where suggestions for different approaches can be made successfully.

In general, families who do not know why they are in early intervention need to be supported through the first few visits, until they like the home visitor, even if they cannot identify why he or she comes to the home!

Families with Multiple or Complex Needs

Home visitors who are used to dealing primarily with developmental skills can sometimes be overwhelmed when families have multiple or complex needs, such as poverty-related stresses, intra- or extrafamilial conflict, or medical needs of the child or other family members. Many home visitors are trained in child-related topics other than medical needs, so these family-related and medical issues are frightening in their unfamiliarity, chronicity, and severity. On home visits to such families, it might be helpful to ask all the other questions before Question 3 on the VHVS to ensure the family's priorities are addressed. This helps prevent regression to the familiar by the home visitor who might be more comfortable with child outcomes. If the IFSP had been done well, of course, the IFSP would address these complex needs.

Families Who Want More Than We Have to Offer

Particularly challenging are families who want many services and lots of them. Early intervention programs might not offer that level of service either because of capacity or because of a different interpretation of how children learn and how services work. Families who believe that more is better (McWilliam, Young, & Harville, 1996) might attribute child progress to periodic (e.g., weekly) services, rather than the ongoing interactions the child has with the environment. It is understandable, then, that they might think that the child should get as many of these services as possible. They presumably correctly interpret 1 or 2 hours a week of *intervention* as insufficient for a child. Unfortunately, the level of *service* a child would need would be so huge to make a difference in his or her learning and development (e.g., perhaps 15 hours a week or more), that that level of service would be unattainable through home visits. If early interventionists are unsuccessful in explaining to families that home visits are designed to prepare natural caregivers for all the time between home visits, those families might be better served through a group-care program, where the child will have other adults involved for enough hours in the day to have a direct impact. Therefore, home visitors working with families wanting many hours of service should, first, attempt to explain to families how children learn and how services work and, second, suggest to families that group care might be an option. They should not blindly apply more services, which can do harm: It can teach families that young children learn from massed trials out of context. It is more supportive of families to teach them that children learn through dispersed trials in context.

CONCLUSION

To serve families well in home visits, it is recommended that professionals

- Use accessible materials rather than a toy bag.
- Engage in "kitchen talk," paying attention to all the family needs that affect the child's development, rather than working just with the child.
- Encourage families through emotional support.
- Work on sensible, helpful goals that improve families' satisfaction with their routines (i.e., quality of life) and follow the Vanderbilt Home Visit Script.
- Find out what families want to be shown and model as necessary and deliberately, rather than modeling unnecessarily.
- Talk about everyday routines (what happens *between* home visits) and talk to families, rather than implying that "lessons" or "sessions" are important and "working with" the child.
- Keep the focus on learning opportunities that occur naturally in family routines as opposed to taking early intervention activities and placing them in routines.

REFERENCES

Bailey, D. B., Jr., Aytch, L. S., Odom, S. L., Symons, F., & Wolery, M. (1999). Early intervention as we know it. *Mental Retardation and Developmental Disabilities Research Reviews, 5,* 11–20.

Bruder, M. B. (2000). Family-centered early intervention: Clarifying our values for the new millennium. *Topics in Early Childhood Special Education, 20,* 105–115.

Bruder, M. B., & Dunst, C. J. (2006). Early intervention service coordination models and service coordination practices. *Journal of Early Intervention, 28,* 155–166.

Campbell, P. H. (1987). The integrated programming team: An approach for coordinating professionals of various disciplines in programs for students with severe and multiple handicaps. *Journal of the Association for Persons with Severe Handicaps, 12,* 107–116.

Danielson, L., Doolittle, J., & Bradley, R. (2007). Professional development, capacity building, and research needs: Critical issues for response to intervention implementation. *School Psychology Review, 36,* 632–637.

de Kruif, R. E. L., & McWilliam, R. A. (1999). Multivariate relationships among developmental age, global engagement, and observed child engagement. *Early Childhood Research Quarterly, 14,* 515–536.

Duggan, A., McFarlane, E., Fuddy, L., Burrell, L., Higman, S. M., Windham, A., et al. (2004). Randomized trial of a statewide home visiting program: Impact in preventing child abuse and neglect. *Child Abuse and Neglect, 28,* 597–622.

Dunst, C. J. (1999). Placing parent education in conceptual and empirical context. *Topics in Early Childhood Special Education, 19,* 141–147.

Dunst, C. J. (2001). Participation in community learning activities. In M. J. Guralnick (Ed.), *Early childhood inclusion: Focus on change* (pp. 307–336). Baltimore: Brookes.

Dunst, C. J., Hamby, D., Trivette, C. M., Raab, M., & Bruder, M. B. (2002). Young children's participation in everyday family and community activity. *Psychological Reports, 91,* 875–897.

Dunst, C. J., & McWilliam, R. A. (1988). Cognitive assessment of multiply handicapped young children. In T. D. Wachs & R. Sheehan (Eds.), *Assessment of young developmentally disabled children* (pp. 213–238). New York: Plenum Press.

Dunst, C. J., & Trivette, C. M. (1988). Helping, helplessness and harm. In J. Witt, S. Elliott, & F. Gresham (Eds.), *Handbook of behavior therapy in education* (pp. 343–376). New York: Plenum.

Edelman, L. (2001). *Just being kids: Supports and services for infants and toddlers and their families in everyday routines, activities, and places* [Videotape with facilitator's guide]. Denver, CO: Western Media Products.

Gelfand, D. M., Teti, D. G., Seiner, S. A., & Jameson, B. (1996). Helping mothers fight depression: Evaluation of a home-based intervention program for depressed mothers and their infants. *Journal of Clinical Child Psychology, 25,* 406–422.

Greenwood, C., Walker, D., Bailey, D., & ECO Center Colleagues (2005, October). *Critical issues in measuring outcomes for young children and their families.* Paper presented at the Annual Meeting of the CEC Division for Early Childhood Conference, Portland, OR. Retrieved April 30, 2006, from *www.fpg.unc.edu/~ECO/presentations.cfm.*

Gresham, F. M. (2007). Response to intervention and emotional and behavioral disorders: Best practices in assessment for intervention. *Assessment for Effective Intervention, 32,* 214–222.

Grisham-Brown, J. C., Schuster, J. W. C., Hemmeter, M. L. C., & Collins, B. C. (2000). Using an embedding strategy to teach preschoolers with significant disabilities. *Journal of Behavioral Education, 10,* 139–162.

Guralnick, M. J. (1998). Effectiveness of early intervention for vulnerable children: A developmental perspective. *American Journal on Mental Retardation, 102,* 319–345.

Guralnick, M. J. (2001). A framework for change in early childhood inclusion. In M. J. Guralnick (Ed.), *Early childhood inclusion: Focus on change* (pp. 3–38). Baltimore: Brookes.

Hanft, B. E., & Feinberg, E. (1997). Toward the development of a framework for determining the frequency and intensity of early intervention services. *Infants and Young Children, 10,* 27–37.

Hanft, B. E., Rush, D. D., & Shelden, M. L. (2004). *Coaching families and colleagues in early childhood.* Baltimore: Brookes.

Harbin, G. L. (2005). Designing an integrated point of access in the early intervention system. In M. J. Guralnick (Ed.), *The developmental systems approach to early intervention* (pp. 99–132). Baltimore: Brookes.

Hart, B., & Risley, T. R. (1974). Using preschool materials to modify the language of disadvantaged children. *Journal of Applied Behavior Analysis, 7,* 243–256.

Hart, B., & Risley, T. R. (1975). Incidental teaching of language in the preschool. *Journal of Applied Behavior Analysis, 8,* 411–420.

Horner, R. H., Dunlap, G., & Koegel, R. L. (Eds.). (1988). *Generalization and maintenance: Lifestyle changes in applied settings.* Baltimore: Brookes.

Jung, L. A., & McWilliam, R. A. (2005). Reliability and validity of scores on the IFSP Rating Scale. *Journal of Early Intervention, 27,* 125–136.

Kaiser, A., Mahoney, G., Girolametto, L., MacDonald, J., Robinson, C., Safford, P., et al. (1999). Rejoinder: Toward a contemporary vision of parent education. *Topics in Early Childhood Special Education, 19,* 173–176.

Kendrick, D., Elkan, R., Hewitt, M., Dewey, M., Blair, M., Robinson, J., et al. (2000). Does home visiting improve parenting and the quality of the home environment? A systematic review and meta analyis. *Archives of Disease in Childhood, 82,* 443–451.

Korfmacher, J., Kitzman, H., & Olds, D. (1998). Intervention processes as predictors of outcomes in a preventive home-visitation program. *Journal of Community Psychology, 26,* 49–64.

Kratochwill, T. R., Albers, C. A., & Shernoff, E. S. (2004). School-based interventions. *Child and Adolescent Psychiatric Clinics of North America, 13,* 885–903.

Liaw, F., Meisels, S. J., Brooks-Gunn, J. (1995). The effects of experience of early intervention on low birth weight, premature children: The infant health and development program. *Early Childhood Research Quarterly, 10,* 405–431.

Love, J. M., Kisker, E. E., Ross, C., Raikes, H., Constantine, J., Boller, K., et al. (2005). The effectiveness of Early Head Start for 3-year-old children and their parents: Lessons for policy and programs. *Developmental Psychology, 41,* 885–901.

Mahoney, G., Kaiser, A., Girolametto, L., MacDonald, J., Robinson, C., Safford, P., et al. (1999). Parent education in early intervention: A call for a renewed focus. *Topics in Early Childhood Special Education, 19,* 131–140.

McBride, S. L., & Peterson, C. (1997). Home-based early intervention with families of children with disabilities: Who is doing what? *Topics in Early Childhood Special Education, 17,* 209–233.

McIntyre, L. L., & Phaneuf, L. K. (2007). A three-tier model of parent education in early childhood: Applying a problem-solving model. *Topics in Early Childhood Special Education, 27,* 214–222.

McWilliam, R. A. (1992). *Family-centered intervention planning: A routines-based approach.* Tucson, AZ: Communication Skill Builders.

McWilliam, R. A. (1998). *The rules: Family-centered practices in different early intervention service delivery models.* Georgia Association on Young Children 32nd Annual Conference, "Natural Environments: Interventions Where They Count" [featured speaker], October 9, 1998, Atlanta, GA.

McWilliam, R. A. (2000). It's only natural . . . to have early intervention in the environments where it's needed. In S. Sandall & M. Ostrosky (Eds.), *Young exceptional children monograph series no. 2: Natural environments and inclusion* (pp. 17–26). Denver, CO: Division for Early Childhood of the Council for Exceptional Children.

McWilliam, R. A. (2002, June). *Support-based home visits.* Paper presented at the annual meeting of the National Early Intervention Association. Coimbra, Portugal.

McWilliam, R. A. (2003). Giving families a chance to talk so they can plan. *News Exchange* [newsletter of the American Association for Home-Based Early Intervention], *8*(3), 1, 4–6.

McWilliam, R. A. (2004). *Vanderbilt home visit script.* Center for Child Development, Vanderbilt University Medical Center, Nashville, TN.

McWilliam, R. A. (2005a). Assessing the resource needs of families in the context of early intervention. In M. J. Guralnick (Ed.), *A developmental systems approach to early intervention* (pp. 215–234). Baltimore: Brookes.

McWilliam, R. A. (2005b). *Satisfaction with Home Routines Evaluation (SHoRE).* Vanderbilt University Medical Center, Nashville, TN. Availab;e at *www.siskin.org.*

McWilliam, R. A. (2006). *RBI report form.* Vanderbilt University Medical Center, Nashville, TN. Available at *www.VanderbiltChildrens.org/childdevelopment/.*

McWilliam, R. A., & Bailey, D. B. (1992). Promoting engagement and mastery. In D. B. Bailey & M. Wolery (Eds.), *Teaching infants and preschoolers with disabilities* (2nd ed., pp. 229–256). Columbus, OH: Merrill.

McWilliam, R. A., & Scott, S. (2001). A support approach to early intervention: A three-part framework. *Infants and Young Children, 13*(4), 55–66.

McWilliam, R. A., Snyder, P., Harbin, G. L., Porter, P., & Munn, D. (2000). Professionals' and families' perceptions of family-centered practices in infant-toddler services. *Early Education and Development, 11,* 519–538.

McWilliam, R. A., Tocci, L., & Harbin, G. L. (1998). Family-centered services: Service providers' discourse and behavior. *Topics in Early Childhood Special Education, 18,* 206–221.

McWilliam, R. A., Wolery, M., & Odom, S. L. (2001). Instructional perspectives in inclusive preschool classrooms. In M. J. Guralnick (Ed.), *Early childhood inclusion: Focus on change* (pp. 503–530). Baltimore: Brookes.

McWilliam, R. A., Young, H. J., & Harville, K. (1996). Therapy services in early intervention: Current status, barriers, and recommendations. *Topics in Early Childhood Special Education, 16,* 348–374.

Park, J., Hoffman, L., Marquis, J., Turnbull, A. P., Poston, D. J., Mannan, H., et al. (2003). Toward assessing family outcomes of service delivery: Validation of a family quality of life survey. *Journal of Intellectual Disability Research, 47,* 367–384.

Park, J., Turnbull, A. P., & Turnbull, H. R. (2002). Impacts of poverty on quality of life in families of children with disabilities. *Exceptional Children, 68,* 151–170.

Powell, D. (1993). Inside home visiting programs. *The Future of Children, 3*(3), 1–16.

Premack, D. (1959). Toward empirical behavior laws: I. Positive reinforcement. *Psychological Review, 66,* 219–233.

Risley, T. R., & Cataldo, M. F. (1973). *Planned activity check: Materials for training observers.* Lawrence, KS: Center for Applied Behavior Analysis.

Roberts, R. N., Rule, S., & Innocenti, M. S. (1998). Strengthening the family–professional partnership in services for young children. Baltimore: Brookes.

United States Department of Education. (2003). *Twenty-fifth annual report to Congress on the implementation of the Individuals with Disabilities Education Act.* Washington, DC: Author.

Wolery, M., Anthony, L., Caldwell, N. K., Snyder, E. D., & Morgante, J. D. (2002). Embedding and distributing constant time delay in circle time and transitions. *Topics in Early Childhood Special Education, 22,* 14–25.

Woods, J. J., & Wetherby, A. M. (2003). Early identification of and intervention for infants and toddlers who are at risk for autism spectrum disorder. *Language, Speech, and Hearing Services in Schools, 34,* 180–193.

World Health Organization. (2007). *International classification of functioning, disability and health: Children and youth version icf-cy.* Geneva: WHO Press.

Support-Based Home-Visiting Checklist

Home Visitor: _____ Date: _____

Observer: _____

Did the home visitor . . .	✓ ✗ ? NA	Notes
Emotional support		
1. Make positive statements about the child?		
2. Make positive statements about the adult family members?		
3. Respond to the family's overt or covert requests?		
4. Show concern for family members other than the target child (see also 21)?		
5. Treat the family in a friendly manner, as one would treat a neighbor?		
6. Demonstrate sensitivity to the family's situation?		
The visit		
7. When appropriate, provide information about how to do something with the child?		
8. Provide information about what to do with the child in the context of discussing regular routines?		
9. Consistently listen to the family?		

(cont.)

✓ = done at a satisfactory level; ✗ = not done; ? = perhaps done or done, but perhaps not at a satisfactory level; NA = not appropriate (e.g., ran out of time).

Did the home visitor . . .	✓ ✗ ? NA	Notes
10. Consistently ask questions (rather than just provide information)?		
11. Consistently emphathize?		
12. Consistently encourage the family?		
13. Appropriately offer information to help with a concern?		
14. Appropriately ask whether the concern needed solving (e.g., "Should we try to solve this?")?		
15. Appropriately offer to show the family a technique (instead of not showing or showing without asking)?		
The script		
16. Ask an open-ended opening question to give the family an opportunity to set the agenda for the visit (e.g., "How have things been going?")?		
17. Ask the family whether they have anything new they want to discuss?		
18. Ask the family how things have been going with each of the outcomes or goals on the individualized plan?		
19. Ask the family about outcomes or goals in the family's priority order of importance?		
20. If time, ask the family whether there is a time of day that's not going well for them?		
21. If time, ask about family members other than the child (see also 4)?		
22. If time, ask about any appointments since the previous visit or before the next visit?		
23. If time, ask whether the family has enough or too much to do with the child?		

Vanderbilt Home Visit Script

Directions

The purpose of the Home Visit Script is to give home visitors in early intervention a structure for providing support-based home visits, attending to functional needs of families and the children in those families. It supports professionals in using an alternative to a hands-on, activity-based approach (i.e., "the toy-bag approach") that implies that the visitor is directly helping the child's development. The script instead gives the home visitor a guide for talking to the family about the many dimensions of child and family life that are part of early intervention in natural environments.

The process is applicable for all disciplines—for professionals from all backgrounds who are providing comprehensive home visits. Such home visits are generally conducted by professionals serving in a primary service provider, primary coach, or transdisciplinary role. Professionals who make discipline-specific home visits (e.g., a physical therapist providing physical therapy only during home visits) might need to adapt the script. The script is very applicable for service coordinators.

Throughout the home visit, the home visitor should provide the following evidence-based emotional support (McWilliam, Tocci, & Harbin, 1998):

- Positiveness about the child and other family members.
- Responsiveness to family's overt or covert requests.
- Orientation to the whole family, especially the well-being of the primary caregiver.
- Friendliness: Treat the family as you would treat neighbors.
- Sensitivity: Walk in the family's shoes.

At any time in the home visit, it is likely that it will be appropriate to stop and provide information about how to do something with the child (in the context of discussing regular routines, of course), as prompted in the script.

Script Overview

1. How have things been going?
2. Do you have anything new you want to ask me about?
3. How have things been going with each IFSP outcome, in priority order?
4. Is there a time of day that's not going well for you?
5. How is [family member] doing?
6. Have you had any appointments in the past week? Any coming up?
7. Do you have enough or too much to do with [your child]?

General Well-Being

1. **How have things been going?**
   The opening question is open ended to give the family an opportunity to set the agenda for the visit.

Notes

   (cont.)

Follow-Up Prompts

1. The four E's: Ears (listen), Elicit (ask), Empathize, Encourage
2. *Do you need any information to help with this?*
3. *Should we try to solve this?*
4. *Would you like me to show you?*

New Questions or Concerns

2. Do you have anything new you want to ask me about?

This question is a little more specific, giving the family an opportunity to think about new issues, skills, problems, and so on.

Follow-Up Prompts

1. The four E's: Ears (listen), Elicit (ask), Empathize, Encourage
2. *Do you need any information to help with this?*
3. *Should we try to solve this?*
4. *Would you like me to show you?*

Notes

Outcomes in Priority Order

The outcomes should be functional needs the family has identified. This is best accomplished through some form of routines-based assessment, such as the Routines-Based Interview (McWilliam, 1992), instead of or in addition to developmental assessment. This type of assessment tends to result in 6–10 quite specific, functional, child and family outcomes. It is helpful to have families put their outcomes in priority order. Child outcomes are always discussed in the context of routines.

3. How have things been going with [Priority No. 1]?
Discuss this in the context of routines.

Follow-Up Prompts

1. The four E's: Ears (listen), Elicit (ask), Empathize, Encourage
2. *Do you need any information to help with this?*
3. *Should we try to solve this?*
4. *Would you like me to show you?*

Notes

How have things been going with [Priority No. 2]?

Discuss this in the context of routines.

Follow-Up Prompts

1. The four E's: Ears (listen), Elicit (ask), Empathize, Encourage
2. *Do you need any information to help with this?*
3. *Should we try to solve this?*
4. *Would you like me to show you?*

Notes

How have things been going with [Priority No. 3]?

Discuss this in the context of routines.

(cont.)

Follow-Up Prompts
1. The four E's: Ears (listen), Elicit (ask), Empathize, Encourage
2. *Do you need any information to help with this?*
3. *Should we try to solve this?*
4. *Would you like me to show you?*

Notes

How have things been going with [Priority No. 4]?

Discuss this in the context of routines.

Notes

Follow-Up Prompts
1. The four E's: Ears (listen), Elicit (ask), Empathize, Encourage
2. *Do you need any information to help with this?*
3. *Should we try to solve this?*
4. *Would you like me to show you?*

How have things been going with [Priority No. 5]?

Discuss this in the context of routines.

Notes

Follow-Up Prompts
1. The four E's: Ears (listen), Elicit (ask), Empathize, Encourage
2. *Do you need any information to help with this?*
3. *Should we try to solve this?*
4. *Would you like me to show you?*

How have things been going with [Priority No. 6]?

Discuss this in the context of routines.

Notes

Follow-Up Prompts
1. The four E's: Ears (listen), Elicit (ask), Empathize, Encourage
2. *Do you need any information to help with this?*
3. *Should we try to solve this?*
4. *Would you like me to show you?*

How have things been going with [Priority No. 7]?

Discuss this in the context of routines.

Notes

Follow-Up Prompts
1. The four E's: Ears (listen), Elicit (ask), Empathize, Encourage
2. *Do you need any information to help with this?*
3. *Should we try to solve this?*
4. *Would you like me to show you?*

How have things been going with [Priority No. 8]?

Discuss this in the context of routines.

Notes

Follow-Up Prompts
1. The four E's: Ears (listen), Elicit (ask), Empathize, Encourage
2. *Do you need any information to help with this?*
3. *Should we try to solve this?*
4. *Would you like me to show you?*

(cont.)

Problematic Routines

4. Is there a time of day that's not going well for you?

This question provides the family an opportunity to discuss a routine that continues to be or has become unsatisfactory.

Follow-Up Prompts

1. The four E's: Ears (listen), Elicit (ask), Empathize, Encourage
2. *Do you need any information to help with this?*
3. *Should we try to solve this?*
4. *Would you like me to show you?*

Notes

Other Family Members

5. How is [family member] doing?

This question reinforces to the family that you understand that the child lives in the context of a whole family.

Follow-Up Prompts

1. The four E's: Ears (listen), Elicit (ask), Empathize, Encourage
2. *Do you need any information to help with this?*
3. *Should we try to solve this?*
4. *Would you like me to show you?*

Notes

Appointments

6. Have you had any appointments in the past week? Any coming up?

These questions help the family organize the information they receive from other professionals and questions they might want to ask other professionals.

Follow-Up Prompts

1. The four E's: Ears (listen), Elicit (ask), Empathize, Encourage
2. *Do you need any information to help with this?*
3. *Should we try to solve this?*
4. *Would you like me to show you?*

Notes

Work Load Related to Intervention

7. Do you have enough or too much to do with [your child]?

This question demonstrates your sensitivity and responsiveness.

Follow-Up Prompts

1. The four E's: Ears (listen), Elicit (ask), Empathize, Encourage
2. *Do you need any information to help with this?*
3. *Should we try to solve this?*
4. *Would you like me to show you?*

Notes

CHAPTER 9

Helping Families
Address Challenging Behavior
and Promote Social Development

LISE FOX

As very young children develop, problem behaviors are expected. This chapter is focused on assisting young children with disabilities whose problem behaviors exceed what is developmentally expected, persist in ways that are not normative, or are of the intensity or frequency that is not typical of most young children. It provides home visitors with information on understanding challenging behavior and its impact on the family and how to guide families in effectively responding to the needs of their child with developmental delays and challenging behavior.

Children who have not developed a sophisticated repertoire of communication and social skills to express their needs, protest actions and events, and gain attention use problem behaviors such as whining, crying, aggression, tantrums, biting, and noncompliance (Powell, Dunlap, & Fox, 2006). As children grow older and develop conventional and socially acceptable ways to communicate and learn social skills, these behaviors begin to diminish. In contrast, challenging behaviors are more intensive (e.g., tantrums of long duration), more frequent, or more severe (e.g., self-injury) than developmentally expected behaviors. Challenging severe behaviors might not diminish with age and often continue to intensify in frequency and severity.

Research indicates that problem behaviors identified in the preschool years have a high likelihood of persisting into adolescence and adulthood (Dunlap, Strain, et. al., 2006). Teenagers described as emotionally disturbed have a history of problem behavior as far back as the preschool years (Campbell & Ewing, 1990; Loeber & Dishion, 1983; Moffitt, Caspi, Dickson, Silva, & Stanton, 1996). Problem

237

behaviors identified in preschool are stable and continue to be present 3–7 years later (Campbell, 1995; Campbell & Ewing, 1990; Egeland, Kalkoske, Gottesman, & Erickson, 1990; Fischer, Rolf, Hasazi, & Cummings, 1984; Lavigne et al., 1998; Moreland & Dumas, 2008; Richman, Stevenson, & Graham, 1982; Shaw, Gilliom, & Giovannelli, 2000).

An examination of the impact and outcomes of challenging behavior shows that children and students with disabilities are particularly at risk for difficulties. A longitudinal study of students in special education found that problem behaviors were quite common among students with disabilities (United States Department of Education [USDOE], 2002). Mild problem behaviors such as distractibility and impulsivity were the most prevalent problem behaviors (38% and 25%, respectively), with aggression and isolation reported less frequently (6.9% and 9.8%, respectively). Students with disabilities have more than three times the number of serious misconduct incidents per 1,000 students than do typically developing students (United States General Accounting Office [GAO], 2001). About 50% of students identified with emotional and behavioral disorders drop out of school, leading to poor job outcomes, limited income, and a pattern of failure that persists into adulthood (USDOE, 2001). These problems are evident in even the youngest children served by the Individuals with Disabilities Education Act (IDEA). Data from the National Early Intervention Longitudinal Study (NEILS), tracking infants and toddlers served by IDEA Part C, indicate that 10–40% of the children are described as having behavioral challenges (USDOE, 2001). Those behavior challenges range from excitable and very active (39%) to aggressive (11%).

THE EFFECT OF CHALLENGING BEHAVIOR ON THE FAMILY

Challenging behavior affects the whole family's quality of life, including the child's. Young children with challenging behavior can experience expulsions from early childhood programs (Gilliam, 2005), restricted access to activities and environments frequented by young children, and difficulties in play with peers (Lucyshyn, Horner, Dunlap, Albin, & Ben, 2002). When children have challenging behavior, family life is often negatively affected. Parents report that the presence of challenging behavior can affect the entire family system, with stressors to (1) the marriage, (2) access to activities, (3) the ability to parent effectively, and (4) access to social support (Duda, Clarke, Fox, & Dunlap, 2008; Fox, Vaughn, Wyatte, & Dunlap, 2002; Lucyshyn, Kayser, Irvin, & Blumberg, 2002; Turnbull & Ruef, 1996, 1997; Worcester, Nesman, Mendez, & Keller, 2008). For example, families have reported that they have discontinued attending church, are reluctant to visit friends and family, and do not invite others to their home (Fox, Benito, & Dunlap, 2002; Worcester et al., 2008). Families have reported that their child's challenging behavior leaves them exhausted, frustrated, feeling out of control of their lives, and socially isolated (Fox, Vaughn, et al., 2002).

The stress that challenging behavior contributes to the family system is an important consideration while the professional provides support and guidance to the family. Consider the following example of how challenging behavior affects the entire family:

Danny is a 2 year old with autism who has many severe behavior problems. He lives with his mother, father, and 7-year-old sister, Aimee. He has frequent temper tantrums, as many as 10 a day, that can last from 20 minutes to 2 hours. When he tantrums, he can escalate to the point where he bangs his head on the floor or other hard surfaces (e.g., corner of bed, door frame). Danny also sleeps very erratically and is often up in the night wandering around the house. When his mother tries to put him to bed, it triggers a tantrum. As a consequence, his mother is resigned to staying awake to watch him. Danny's mother has withdrawn him from preschool because she fears that the teachers are unable to manage his behavior. She is also frightened to leave him at home with a child care provider. As a consequence, Aimee has withdrawn from the soccer league and her Brownie troop. Her mother is unable to manage Danny and drive her daughter to those events. Danny's mother has suggested that Aimee bring friends over to play at her house, but Aimee rejects the idea. Aimee often asks to go to the park, library, or store. Her mother responds that it is not possible to handle Danny in those settings. When Danny's father comes home in the evenings, he can see the tension and exhaustion and feels frustrated in his efforts to make it better for everyone.

The kind of stress that is occurring in Danny's family begins to affect all family members and their emotional well-being. When working with the family around a child's problem behavior, it will be important to recognize the stressors the behavior puts on the family and be able to provide guidance that is focused on supporting the family unit as well as the individual child.

A FRAMEWORK FOR PROVIDING SUPPORT

As early childhood special educators consider their support of families whose children have challenging behavior, it is particularly important to realize that the notion of what is challenging behavior is culturally defined. Families have unique and idiosyncratic perspectives about what behaviors might be accepted or tolerated (Cheatham & Santos, 2005; Chen, Downing, & Peckham-Hardin, 2002). When supporting families around behavior issues, it will be important to acknowledge that there can be cultural differences that will affect the topics families are comfortable discussing, the identification of priorities or needs regarding the child's behavior, the social acceptance of various discipline and behavior intervention practices, and the assessment of meaningful outcomes (Barrera & Corso, 2003).

The approach to helping families address challenging behavior discussed in this chapter is based upon some important assumptions. First, young children engage in challenging behavior because it serves a purpose for them. This does not mean that children make a decision to engage in challenging behavior; rather, their challenging behavior results in an effect or response from an adult or peer that meets the child's need. In this manner, problem behavior can be viewed as purposeful. A related assumption is that the child persists in using problem behavior because it "works" for him or her. When young children use problem behavior it typically results in gaining access or escaping an object, activity, or attention (Nielsen, Olive, Donovan, & McEvoy, 1998; O'Neill, Vaughn, & Dunlap, 1998). The final assumption is that when young children use challenging behavior to get their needs met, the most effective intervention is to teach the child replacement social and emotional skills.

INITIATING THE CONVERSATION

In early intervention programs, the professional's role is to support the family in identifying the social and communication skills that can be taught to the child to replace problem behavior and in promoting the child's acquisition and fluent use of those skills. Thus, the early interventionist must be able to work collaboratively with family members to promote their capacity to support the child.

In this chapter, guidance is provided on how to begin conversations with families about their concerns about their child's behavior, how to provide information on positive parenting techniques, and how to help families plan and implement support strategies for children with developmental delays and persistent problem behavior. Appendix 9.1 at the end of this chapter provides the professional with suggestions on how to initiate and respond to family concerns about challenging behavior.

Understanding Family Concerns

Initiating a discussion about a child's challenging behavior is a sensitive undertaking. Many families report that they feel judged by others as being bad or neglectful parents and are reluctant to ask for assistance for their child's behavior. The early interventionist must initiate the conversation with care and with sensitivity to the family's approachability on the issue. The following examples provide illustrations of initiating the topic of providing guidance on problem behavior, by empathizing with the family member and offering support.

Ms. Rafael mentioned that her son had been asked to leave his child care center because he was having problem behavior. Emily, her early interventionist, noted the comment and said, "That must be disappointing to you. I know you need child care in the afternoons. Tell me more about what some of his behaviors were. I'd like to offer to help you figure out how to help him learn new behaviors so that this doesn't happen again."

Ben was conducting a home visit with Mrs. Charles, the grandmother of Kara, who was sitting in her grandmother's lap, bouncing up and down. Mrs. Charles put her hand on her thigh and asked her to stop. Kara leaned down and bit her grandmother's arm. Mrs. Charles slapped her face and reprimanded her by saying, "You are a bad girl, don't you bite! Get off me." Kara jumped off her grandmother's lap and ran out of the room. Ben asked Mrs. Charles about the bite: "Are you OK?" And then he said, "That must have hurt. Often children Kara's age bite . . . it's not OK . . . but it is pretty common."

Mrs. Charles responded with "She just doesn't mind me."

Ben replied, "I can see that Kara is difficult to manage and I know you want to make sure she learns right from wrong. If you would like me to, I can give you some suggestions for how to help her learn to follow your instructions."

When initiating the conversation about challenging behavior with family members, it is important that the early interventionist receives information from the family without expressing alarm or judgment. It will be important that the family see the early interventionist as an ally and a support to them in their role as parents. If the early interventionist reacts to the sharing of information by visibly showing disapproval or shock at the information, the family is unlikely to continue to share information or ask for support. When families begin to open up with concerns about the child's behavior, the early interventionist can gain important information that will help in developing an understanding of the behavior and behavior support needs by asking the following questions:

1. What are the behaviors that are most problematic?
2. What have you tried to do to resolve these behaviors?
3. What routines or activities are most difficult because of the behaviors?

As family members respond to these questions, the early interventionist should receive the information with empathy and reassurance. When discussing the topic of problem behavior with families, the interventionist can find that his or her personal values about child discipline, parenting practices, and family history of being parented might influence the interventionist's reactions or perspectives about what families will divulge. It is critically important that the interventionist remain objective, open, and willing to offer support to families. If a professional's biases on this topic become evident, the families they want to support are not likely to reveal this kind of very personal and emotional information. Consider the two examples below. Ben listens to Mrs. Perez share her concerns about Maria's behavior and offers reassurance, acknowledges the parent's strengths, and is able to gain her interest in learning support strategies. The other example illustrates the struggle that Katie has in separating her reaction to what Ms. Clarke has shared from what she should do.

> Mrs. Perez has asked Ben for advice about her daughter Maria's behavior. She shared with him that Maria is out of control with her tantrums. Maria will hit, scratch, bite, throw toys, and try to vomit when she is upset. Mrs. Perez expressed that she has run out of ideas of what to do. Ben asked gently, "Tell me what you do when she has the tantrum." Mrs. Perez responded, "I don't know what to do. Last night she had a tantrum while I was making dinner and I just put her in her room and locked the door. We put a lock on the outside of her door. She stayed in there until morning. I just couldn't deal with her."
>
> Ben touched Mrs. Perez's hand reassuringly and said, "It sounds like you are very frustrated. I think I can help you figure some of this out."

> Katie is talking to Ms. Clarke about Joey's problem behavior. Ms. Clarke told her that Joey had urinated in his sister's bed because he was angry with her. Katie asked Ms. Clarke how she responded to the incident. Ms. Clarke told her, "I was so mad; I did what my Momma would have done to me. I told him if he ruined his sister's bed, he didn't deserve to have a bed. I made him sleep on the floor for the rest of the week. He sure didn't like that." Katie's eyes opened wide and her expression became alarmed. She did not know what to say and did not respond. Ms. Perez continued, "So, you think I am a bad Momma, don't you? I tell you, this child is out of control and just needs more of that kind of discipline."

Educators who are primarily involved in providing children with center-based early education programs often find the initiation of a discussion about problem behavior particularly challenging. Table 9.1 provides some guidance on how to talk to families when there is a concern about a child's challenging behavior. The discussion with families about concerns is always a bit difficult. These discussions are easier to have however, when the professional has fostered a trusting relationship with the family and the family views the professional as motivated by a desire to support the child and family.

Addressing Discipline Techniques

One topic that is difficult for interventionists to address is the use of discipline techniques that are harsh or inappropriate. The early interventionist should address these concerns, but carefully. The goal of a conversation with a family member about discipline techniques is to provide the family with effective alternatives that will promote the child's development. This conversation should be devoid of judgment or corrective feedback. Consider the example of how Michelle was able to initiate a conversation about the use of spanking in a manner that expressed support to the parent.

TABLE 9.1. Talking with Families about Problem Behavior: Dos and Don'ts

Do	Don't
Begin the discussion by expressing concern about the child.	Begin the discussion by indicating that the child's behavior is not tolerable.
Let the parent know that your goal is to help the child.	Indicate that the child must be punished or "dealt with" by the parent.
Ask the parent whether he or she has experienced similar situations and are concerned.	Ask the parent whether something has happened at home to cause the behavior.
Tell the parent that you want to work with the family to help the child develop appropriate behavior and social skills.	Indicate that the parent should take action to resolve the problem at home.
Tell the parent about what is happening in the classroom but only after the parent understands that you are concerned about the child, not blaming the family.	Initiate the conversation by listing the child's problem behavior. Discussions about problem behavior should be framed as "the child is having a difficult time," rather than losing control.
Offer to work with the parent in the development of a behavior support plan that can be used at home and in the classroom.	Leave it up to the parent to manage problems at home; develop a plan without inviting family participation.
Emphasize that your focus will be to help the child develop the skills needed to be successful in the classroom.	Let the parent believe that the child needs more discipline. The child needs instruction and support.

Michelle arrived for a home visit and noticed a man's belt hanging from a hook in the hall. The mother said the belt was for disciplining the children. Michelle asked, "Do you have to use the belt often?" The mother responded that the last time she used it was for her 7-year-old, because he stole money from a friend. She confided in Michelle, "I think the belt is a good reminder for them to behave; they know what will happen when they don't." Michelle said, "One thing I would like to do as we work together is continue to talk about some of the problem behaviors your children might have and help you think of ways to teach them to behave appropriately. I know you don't like having to use the belt."

In addressing discipline techniques, some families will need information on child development and guidance on what can be expected from their child. The parent might find a handout on developmental milestones for social development and adaptive behavior to be helpful. In addition, the early interventionist can initiate conversations with the family about what can be expected of young children, especially if the family expects the child to comply with requests or expectations that are not developmentally appropriate. A good way to start this conversation might be in this manner: "Because Katelyn is 3, I want to talk with you about what we can expect 3-year-olds to do, and that way you will be able to challenge her but not have expectations that will frustrate her." In addition, the early interventionist might have to encourage a family member to raise his or her expectations and support the child's development of social skills and independent behavior. Keep in mind that all of this advice must be filtered through knowledge of the family and child's culture and values (Barrera & Corso, 2003). The early interventionist should be cautious to not provide information to the family that reflects his or her own value system or cultural expectations that might be at odds with the family's.

Although some families might have a history of using harsh discipline practices, the early interventionist should guide the family to consider alternative techniques that are positive and focused on supporting the child to learn appropriate behavior and social skills. One strategy for helping the family examine their discipline practices is to pose a question about what new skills are being taught to the child when they use spanking or other harsh punishment practices. The parent might respond that the child is learning the rule or learning to follow the adult's directions. The early interventionist's response should be to acknowledge the parent's perspective and ask again if the discipline technique teaches the child "what to do." Often, that conversation can help families reconsider their approach to discipline. Another way to guide families to reconsider a discipline technique is to ask the family if they believe the technique is working or if the child is getting better. If they respond that the child does not seem to be responding and they are still experiencing problem behavior, the early interventionist can suggest that the family consider another approach.

PROVIDING INFORMATION ON POSITIVE PARENTING TECHNIQUES

When working with families on issues of challenging behavior, many behavior issues might be resolved by teaching the parents some explicit strategies for teaching their child appropriate behavior and establishing expectations. Families might not know how to use these approaches or need additional support in how to use these techniques with their child who has developmental delays.

Two of the most powerful parenting techniques that can be taught to a family are the use of *specific praise* and *stating expectations positively*. Unfortunately, when families are faced with problem behavior, they often get caught in an endless cycle of telling the child "Stop," "Don't" and "No," without providing the child with guidance about what is expected or what the child should do. In addition, often, families are so frustrated by the problem behavior that they have ceased to provide the child with specific praise for behaviors they would like to strengthen. The use of specific, contingent praise is a strategy that is critical to supporting the child's appropriate behavior. Parents frequently overlook the importance of using praise to increase desired behaviors and decrease unwanted behaviors. A lack of praise, however, can lead to inappropriate behavior and fewer positive behaviors. Praise takes very little time and is a very effective way to promote positive behaviors. While some families could be responsive to guidance to "catch the child being good," it might be more meaningful to point out the circumstances where family members naturally use praise and comment on the power of its use. In the following example, Amanda provides Sammi's mother with feedback that encourages her to continue the use of praise.

> "I was watching Sammi while you played with him. Every time you said something like, 'Look at you, you are working so hard,' or, 'I am so proud of the way you are sitting in your chair,' he smiled and tried harder. I think giving him that kind of encouragement really motivates him to learn."

When guiding families to use praise, the early interventionist should consider not only the content of the statement or action but also the way praise is delivered. Suggestions for the delivery of praise in a manner that will have an impact are to (1) gain the child's attention; (2) use behavior-specific language (e.g., state what the child did); (3) avoid combining a praise statement with a criticism; (4) praise with enthusiasm; (5) double the impact with physical warmth (e.g., hug, touch, high-five the child); and (6) praise the child in front of others.

The second powerful parenting technique, stating expectations positively, is one that is critical to providing children with appropriate guidance. For children with special needs, some parents will need information on how to communicate expectations in a manner that children will understand (Mirenda, MacGregor, & Kelly-Keough, 2002). The early interventionist should be ready to provide families with information on how to deliver an instruction in a way that the child understands the parent's expectation. For example, for a child with visual impairments, the early interventionist can show the parent how to use objects paired with a verbal request to help a child transition to a routine, such as handing him or her the soap and then say "Time to wash hands. We wash our hands before eating." Or using pictures to assist the child with autism with moving through the steps of the morning routine, such as getting dressed, eating breakfast, brushing teeth, and getting in the car for preschool.

In addition to expectations for following directions or a routine, families can be encouraged to establish household behavior expectations and begin teaching those expectations to their children. When encouraging families to set household expectations, they should be guided to decide on a small number (three to five) rules that have general applicability to a variety of situations. For example, the rules might be "Tell an adult where you are going," "Clean up," and "Solve problems with words." Families can be encouraged to post their rules, using a format the child can understand (e.g., written with photos of child demonstrating the rule).

Once rules are established, families might also need specific information on how to teach those expectations. Table 9.2 provides some guidance on how one can explain to families instructional strategies for teaching behavior expectations.

TABLE 9.2. Teaching Behavior Expectations

1. *Step by step.* Children will need to have tasks broken down for them. Often we have to help them learn how to do the skill before we can expect them to do it independently. That might involve showing them how, doing part of something, and having them finish it, or asking them to only do a part of the skill.

2. *Review, review, review.* When you learn something new, it can take repeated review of the new information before you really get it. Children are the same way. If you show your child the rules chart only one time and then forget to review it again, and again, and again, they are going to forget what is on it.

3. *Practice, practice, practice.* Anyone who has learned to play an instrument or do a new sport knows that you have to keep practicing. Children will need lots of practice (and encouragement) to learn new skills.

4. *Support, not criticism.* What if you were trying to learn a new dance step and your partner said, "What are you doing? You are really a terrible dancer." How much will you want to keep trying? When we learn something new, we need people to cheer us on.

5. *Celebrate your success.* When your child begins to pay attention to the chart or follow the rule, have a little celebration. It can be as small as a high five, or you might review the chart at dinner and offer a treat for dessert in celebration of your child's success.

A major area for parenting guidance is the use of prevention techniques to reduce the likelihood that the child will have problem behavior. Simple strategies such as providing children with toys to keep them busy when waiting, nutritious snacks to ensure that problem behavior is not triggered by hunger, attempting more difficult routines and activities when the child is well rested, and paying attention to how much the child tolerates activities might be important to give to the parent. In addition, the early interventionist can offer ideas about simple ways that a child could be prepared for an activity that can prevent problem behavior. For example, a child might need a schedule of activities, possibly pictorially represented, so he or she can anticipate what is coming next in the routine. Another child could be helped by reviewing the expectations of a routine or activity immediately prior to engagement (e.g., reminding a child how to play appropriately with other children before entering the playground). Other prevention strategies could be focused on ways the parent can manage the activity so that problem behavior can be avoided. Consider the following example:

> Ms. Alexander has three children under the age of 5. Her 5-year-old daughter is compliant and often helpful to her. When she goes to the grocery store, however, she has difficulty getting her 3-year-old to wait and not run in the parking lot while she gets the 6-month-old baby out of the car. Once everyone is out of the car, she struggles with carrying the baby while chasing the 3-year-old. She discussed her frustration with Gloria. Gloria helped her think through the activity of getting out of the car and how she could use simple strategies to improve the transition from car to grocery store. Gloria's suggestions included parking the car near a vacant shopping cart, bringing the shopping cart to the side of the car before getting the children out of the car, taking the baby in the baby carrier out first and placing him in the cart, and then getting the children

out of the car. She also suggested that Ms. Alexander do her major shopping trip one evening when the children's father was home, so the shopping trips during the week were shorter. Ms. Alexander was so grateful. She felt these were great ideas, but had not ever taken the time to think through doing the routine differently.

The identification of prevention strategies is also linked to understanding why the child is having challenging behavior. This chapter began by stating that children engage in challenging behavior because it works for them and their problem behavior can be interpreted as meaningful or having a message. The goal in a discussion about a child's challenging behavior should be to develop an understanding of why the behavior is occurring. Once the purpose or function of the behavior is determined, more effective preventions and interventions can be developed. Often, simple questions posed to the family such as "Why do you think he is having a hard time with this?" or "What do you think she wants when she is showing this behavior?" will help the family identify the purpose of the behavior. Part of the early interventionist's guidance to the family will be to think first about the *why* of behavior, consider ways to avoid triggering the behavior, or develop ways to respond to the behavior differently.

RESPONDING EFFECTIVELY TO PROBLEM BEHAVIOR

Many families need information on how to respond to problem behavior in a manner that is not coercive or does not reinforce the problem behavior. There are some simple basic techniques that can be helpful for behavior problems that are typical for many children. These strategies are listed in Table 9.3 and described briefly below.

Planned Ignoring

Young children often engage in minor problem behavior such as whining, making noises, taunting others in an effort to gain the attention of the caregiver or peer. If those behaviors are successful in gaining attention (positive or negative), the

TABLE 9.3. Responding to Problem Behavior

1. Use ignoring for attention-seeking behavior.
2. Provide limited, but reasonable choices.
3. Use when–then contingencies.
4. Redirect child to interrupt problem behavior.
5. Use logical consequences.
6. Stay calm.

child learns that the behaviors are effective. This increases the likelihood that the child will continue to use those behaviors to gain attention. In providing support to families, the early interventionist can help the caregiver distinguish between (1) behaviors that are of little consequence and are aimed at gaining access to attention, and (2) behaviors that are more dangerous or disruptive and call for individually designed behavior supports. This conversation will often begin by asking the family why the child might engage in those behaviors and if the behaviors are harmful. When the parent responds that the behavior is to gain attention (e.g., "He just wants me to come in there," "She is doing it to provoke me"), the interventionist should then pose the question about what the child gained when engaging in the behavior. If the family is able to identify that the behavior is about getting access to attention and that the child is successful in the use of those behaviors (i.e., the child actually gets attention when he or she displays the problem behavior), they might be ready to learn how to use selective attention and ignore minor problem behaviors serving to gain attention.

Limited Choices

Providing limited and reasonable choices is an effective way to support the child when he or she is initially difficult within a routine (McCormick, Jolivette, & Ridgley, 2003). For example, the parent can say, "It is time to get dressed. You can choose: Do you want to wear the red dress or the blue skirt?" to a child who is beginning to have a tantrum about getting dressed. The provision of limited choices provides the child with an opportunity for social control within reasonable and adult-established limits.

When–Then Statements

Setting up contingencies or using when–then statements can also be effective in helping children comply with adult directives. A when–then contingency states for the child that something desirable will occur immediately following compliance with the adult's request. For example, the parent could say, "When you pick up your toys, then you can watch television," or, "When you sit in your chair, then you can have a popsicle." These statements are provided to children in a calm manner as statements of facts, rather than communicating anger, punishment, or cajolement.

Redirection

Redirection is another effective response to a child's problem behavior. A parent can interrupt a challenging behavior and redirect a child to another activity, using either physical or verbal redirection. A verbal redirection distracts the child and provides an alternative activity. For example, a child might be trying to gain the attention of a parent who is on the telephone with an important call. Another adult would then say to the child something like, "Hey Ella, let's go upstairs and play with blocks."

Logical Consequences

Logical consequences are consequences that make sense as a response to a challenging behavior because they are related to the behavior in some way. They are an effective alternative to the use of punishment strategies such as reprimands or scolding. They provide children with guidance on how to behave by demonstrating to them the consequences or outcomes of their behavior. Below are a few examples:

- A child throws a block at her sister—so the parent takes the blocks away.
- A brother and sister are fighting—so the parent sends them to play in separate rooms.
- A child persists at dumping water out of the tub—so the parent ends the bath.

The logical consequence should be first presented to the child as a choice using a verbal statement: "If you continue to throw blocks, I will have to put the blocks away." The statement should be delivered calmly, clearly, and respectfully. Logical consequences are appropriate only when a child understands the options provided and can understand the sequence of events if he or she persists in the problem behavior.

Staying Calm

For many families a critically important strategy in the application of any strategy is to stay calm. Responding calmly to problem behavior with a minimum of attention or angry emotion will reduce the risk of strengthening behavior that the parent wants to discourage. In addition, when families remain calm in the face of problem behavior they are more able to think about how they want to respond. It could be appropriate to guide a parent who is likely to respond quickly and angrily to problem behavior to step back and take a deep breath and then think about his or her response, before taking action.

DEVELOPING A BEHAVIOR SUPPORT PLAN

A few children engage in challenging behavior that is persistent despite the use of positive parenting techniques or typical child guidance procedures. For these children, the process of positive behavior support (PBS) can be used to develop an individualized behavior support plan that family members and other caregivers can implement within daily routines (Boulware, Schwartz, & McBride, 1999; Crimmins, Farrell, Smith, & Bailey, 2007; Dunlap & Fox, 1996; Powell et al., 2006). The process of PBS involves the use of functional assessment to develop an individualized behavior support plan that is focused on teaching children skills to replace problem behavior. PBS is recognized as a research-based practice that results in problem behavior reduction, learning new skills, and improvements in the quality of life for individuals with challenging behavior and their families (Bambara & Kern, 2005; Carr et al., 1999; Fox, Dunlap, & Powell, 2002).

The PBS process results in an assessment-based individualized behavior support plan that is designed to be implemented by the persons who interact with the child or individual with challenging behavior. The family is essential to the process as the family will be responsible for the implementation of the behavior support plan. The phases and activities for implementing PBS are described in the following section to provide the early interventionist guidance on how to facilitate the process. More information on how to implement PBS with young children can be found in additional resources (e.g., *www.challengingbehavior.org, www.csefel.uiuc. edu*).

Functional Assessment

PBS begins with functional assessment, which involves gathering information that will lead to an understanding of the "function" or purpose of the challenging behavior (Bambara & Kern, 2005; Harrower, Fox, Dunlap, & Kincaid, 2000; Lucyshyn et al., 2002). It involves clearly defining the challenging behavior, gathering information on the triggers for the behavior, and identifying the maintaining consequences that follow challenging behavior. The functional assessment involves multiple sources of information and perspectives. An interview for gathering information from the people who know the child well and have observed behavior in key settings is often used (Kern, O'Neill, & Starosta, 2005; O'Neill et al., 1997). In addition to the interview, the early interventionist can observe the child within the activities or routines associated with challenging behavior and record the observations by noting the antecedents to the problem behavior and events that followed problem behavior that serve as maintaining consequences. Early interventionists can also provide the family with a method for writing down their observations (again noting antecedents, behaviors, and maintaining consequences) or debrief with the family on a recent behavior incident by guiding the family to identify the antecedents and maintaining consequences linked to the incident.

Behavior Hypotheses

Information is gathered on when problem behavior is occurring, what antecedents trigger problem behavior, and the responses that follow problem behavior that serve as maintaining consequences until the early interventionist feels that there are ample data on which to develop preliminary hypotheses, with the family, about the purpose or function of the problem behavior within contexts. The behavior hypotheses are statements that summarize the common set of antecedents or triggers, how the child reacts, the function or purpose of the behavior, and the maintaining consequences that follow the behavior (Kern, 2005). Below are two examples of behavior hypothesis statements.

Dana will drop to the floor, scream, cry, and throw objects when asked to come to the dinner table, take a bath, brush teeth, and clean-up toys as a way to escape the activity. When this occurs, his parent will give him more time in the preferred activity or occasionally give up on the request.

When Marco's sister joins in his play, Marco will grab toys from her, slap her, and cry to keep her from touching his toys. When this occurs, Marco's mother reprimands Marco and asks his sister to play in another room or with her own toys.

Developing the Support Plan

Once the behavior hypotheses are identified, the early interventionist should work with the family to identify the strategies that can be used in a behavior support plan (Boulware et al., 1999). The behavior support plan is directly linked to each of the behavior hypotheses. There are three parts to the plan that match the distinct elements of the behavior hypotheses (Dunlap & Fox, 1999). First, the plan includes prevention strategies directly linked to the triggers or antecedents listed in the behavior hypotheses. Prevention strategies serve to soften the triggers or change the antecedent conditions so that problem behavior is less likely to occur. In the example of Marco, if the play setting was arranged so that Marco had duplicate toy sets that his sister could use with him, it would reduce his distress in having her play with him, and he would not engage in the challenging behavior. The second part of the plan is replacement skills linked to the function of the problem behavior.

Replacement skills are the new skills that will be taught to the child to replace the use of problem behavior. For example, currently Marco is aggressive with his sister to keep her from touching his toys. Perhaps he should be taught to say, "Don't touch," or "Mine," to signal that he does not want to share. The third part of the plan is new responses to the problem behavior. These new responses are ways to respond to problem behavior so that the behavior does not achieve a payoff or is maintained. In the example of Marco, his mother reacted by asking Marco's sister to leave the area. This serves to pay off Marco for his problem behavior. A new way to respond might be to ask Marco to use his words to ask the sister not to touch or to ask his mom for help. When designing the behavior support plan, it is very likely that the early interventionist will be the person with ideas for strategies. Parent involvement in developing the plan can be promoted by offering the family an array of strategy suggestions and asking them to make a selection of the strategy that sounds like a good fit for their child and family or asking the family for ideas that tap their knowledge of the child. For example, the early interventionist can say, "This activity would be easier if we added some items that Joey prefers. What are characters or toys that Joey really likes, and can we make them a part of bath time?" Once the strategies to be used in the behavior support plan are determined, the interventionist should provide the family with a written behavior support plan that is easy to understand and follow. When the behavior support plan includes strategies that are routine specific, the interventionist might want to develop routine-based support plans or mini-plans that can be used in that environment. For example, the interventionist can put together in a mini-plan the strategies for going shopping or develop a bedtime chart that can be used to remind the caregiver of the strategies to use in the bedtime routine.

Coaching and Modeling

After the development of the behavior support plan, the early interventionist should guide the family with implementation of the plan. A typical approach to assisting families with plan implementation is to review the plan before the routine and then remind the caregiver of the elements of the plan or specific strategies during their interactions with the child (e.g., Dunlap, Ester, Langhans, & Fox, 2006). If necessary, the interventionist can demonstrate the use of a strategy or technique by role playing with the family. For example, the interventionist might ask the parent to take the role of the child who is refusing to sit in the chair when asked to come to the table for a meal. The parent assumes the role of the child and pretends to cry and run away in response to the direction by the interventionist. The interventionist demonstrates the use of concrete language and gestures, a photo of mealtime as an additional prompt, and physical guidance to move the child to the chair. The role play should occur between the early interventionist and the parent, with one of the adults assuming the role of the child who is demonstrating challenging behavior. The early interventionist should avoid assuming the role of intervention agent and demonstrating the use of the plan with the child as the behavior support plan is designed for the parent to implement.

Monitoring Implementation and Outcomes

The final step of the implementation of PBS is to monitor the implementation of the support plan and track child outcomes. The success of the behavior support plan rests entirely on the fidelity with which the family implements the plan. The early interventionist should consider developing a form to leave with the family for recording their success at implementing the plan and evaluating their child's progress. The form should be easy to understand, easy to complete, and quick. Otherwise it will be of little value to a busy caregiver. Rating scales are effective for this purpose. For example, you can list the major steps of the support plan on a chart and have the parent indicate on a 3-point scale if the strategies were 1 = easy, 2 = a little difficult, or 3 = very difficult to implement. The chart might also include a rating for the child's response. For example, the parent could rate the ease of implementing the plan and then rate the child's engagement in the routine in the following manner: 1 = great, very cooperative; 2 = difficult and uncooperative; or 3 = lots of problem behavior. Although these measurement systems lack precision, they will provide the interventionist with an indication that the plan is being implemented, the parents' facility in using the plan, and the effect of the plan on child behavior.

There might be occasions where the family struggles to implement the plan as initially developed. An important concept related to the implementation of a behavior support plan is contextual fit. Contextual fit refers to how well the behavior support strategies fit with family values, circumstances, and capacities (Albin, Lucyshyn, Horner, & Flannery, 1996; Lucyshyn et al., 2002). When behavior support plans are developed with a sole focus on what the interventionist determines is appropriate without regard for family perspectives, considerations, values, and competing demands, the plan that is developed may not work well for the family. Thus, the implementation of a plan rests, in part, on how well the early interventionist teams with the family in the development of the plan.

Another reason that a family may not implement a plan is because the plan is no longer working for the child or was not effective. It will be important for the early interventionist to check in periodically on how well the plan is working, to ask whether any plan components have been dropped or changed, and to address any issues relating to new behavior challenges or increases in behavior. If the challenging behavior is not changed or if new behaviors develop, the plan should be modified or a functional assessment should be conducted to determine whether there are new triggers or maintaining consequences for the behavior.

CONCLUSION

Supporting families to address their child's challenging behavior is of critical importance to the development of the child and the quality of life of the child and family system. It is a complicated endeavor because it requires the support provider to have both (1) deep knowledge of positive parenting practices and behavior intervention approaches, and (2) the ability to establish a trustful relationship with the family. The goal of these efforts should be to provide the family with the knowledge and skills they need to understand the child's behavior, how to promote the child's social development, and how to enhance the child's participation in family life and the community.

REFERENCES

Albin, R., Lucyshyn, J. M., Horner, R. H., & Flannery, K. B. (1996). Contextual fit for behavioral support plans: A model for "goodness of fit." In L. K. Koegel, R. L. Koegel, & G. Dunlap (Eds.), *Positive behavioral support: Including people with difficult behavior in the community* (pp. 81–98). Baltimore: Brookes.

Bambara, L. M., & Kern, L. (2005). *Individualized supports for students with problem behaviors: Designing positive behavior plans.* New York: Guilford Press.

Barrera, I., & Corso, R. M. (2003). *Skilled dialogue: Strategies for responding to cultural diversity in early childhood.* Baltimore: Brookes.

Boulware, G., Schwartz, I., & McBride, B. (1999). Addressing challenging behaviors at home: Working with families to find solutions. *Young Exceptional Children, 3*(1), 21–27.

Campbell, S. B. (1995). Behavior problems in preschool children: A review of recent research. *Journal of Child Psychology and Psychiatry, 36*(1), 113–149.

Campbell, S. B., & Ewing, L. J. (1990). Hard-to-manage preschoolers: Adjustment at age nine and predictors of continuing symptoms. *Journal of Child Psychology and Psychiatry, 31*, 871–889.

Carr, E. G., Horner, R. H., Turnbull, A. P., Marquis, J. G., McLaughlin, D. M., McAtee, M. L., et al. (1999). *Positive behavior support as an approach for dealing with problem behavior in people with developmental disabilities: A research synthesis.* Washington, DC: AAMR.

Cheatham, G. A., & Santos, R. M. (2005). A-B-Cs of bridging home and school expectations for children and families of diverse backgrounds. *Young Exceptional Children, 8*(3), 3–11.

Chen, D., Downing, J. E., & Peckham-Hardin, K. D. (2002). Working with families of diverse cultural and linguistic backgrounds: Considerations for culturally responsive positive behavior support plans. In J. M. Lucyshyn, G. Dunlap, & R. W. Albin (Eds.), *Families and positive behavior support: Addressing problem behavior in family contexts* (pp. 133–154). Baltimore: Brookes.

Crimmins, D., Farrell, A. F., Smith, P. W., & Bailey, A. (2007). *Positive strategies for students with behavior problems.* Baltimore: Brookes

Duda, M., Clarke, S., Fox, L., & Dunlap, G. (2008). Implementation of positive behavior support with a sibling set in the home environment. *Journal of Early Intervention, 30*, 213–236.

Dunlap, G., Ester, T., Langhans, S., & Fox, L. (2006). Functional communication training with toddlers in home environments. *Journal of Early Intervention, 29*, 81–97.

Dunlap, G., & Fox, L. (1996). Early intervention and serious problem behaviors: A comprehensive approach. In L. K. Koegel, R. L. Koegel, & G. Dunlap (Eds.), *Positive behavior support: Including people with difficult behavior in the community* (pp. 31–50). Baltimore: Brookes.

Dunlap, G., & Fox, L. (1999). A demonstration of behavioral support for young children with autism. *Journal of Positive Behavior Interventions, 1*(2), 77–87.

Dunlap, G., Strain, P. S., Fox, L., Carta, J., Conroy, M., Smith, B. J., et al. (2006). Prevention and intervention with young children's challenging behavior: A summary of current knowledge. *Behavioral Disorders, 32*, 29–45.

Egeland, B., Kalkoske, M., Gottesman, N., & Erickson, M. F. (1990). Preschool behavior problems: Stability and factors accounting for change. *Journal of Child Psychology and Psychiatry, 31*, 891–909.

Fischer, M., Rolf, J. E., Hasazi, J. E., & Cummings, L. (1984). Follow-up of a preschool epidemiological sample: Cross-age continuities and predication of later adjustment with internalizing and externalizing dimensions of behavior. *Child Development, 55*, 137–150.

Fox, L., Benito, N., & Dunlap, G. (2002). Early intervention with families of young children with autism spectrum disorder and problem behavior. In J. Lucyshyn, G. Dunlap, & R. Albin (Eds.), *Families and positive behavioral support: Addressing the challenge of problem behavior in family contexts* (pp. 251–270). Baltimore: Brookes.

Fox, L., Dunlap, G., & Powell, D. (2002). Young children with challenging behavior: Issues and consideration for behavior support. *Journal of Positive Behavior Interventions, 4*, 208–217.

Fox, L., Vaughn, B. J., Wyatte, M. L., & Dunlap, G. (2002). "We can't expect other people to understand": Family perspectives on problem behavior. *Exceptional Children, 68*, 437–451.

Gilliam, W. S. (2005). Prekindergarteners left behind: Expulsion rates in state prekindergarten systems. Retrieved July 20, 2005, from *www.fcd-us.org/PDFs/NationalPreKExpulsionPaper03.02_new.pdf*.

Harrower, J. K., Fox, L., Dunlap, G., & Kincaid, D. (2000). Functional Assessment and Comprehensive Early Intervention. *Exceptionalities, 8*, 189–204.

Kern, L. (2005). Developing hypotheses statements. In L. M. Bambara & L. Kern (Eds.), *Individualized supports for students with problem behaviors* (pp. 165–200). New York: Guilford Press.

Kern, L., O'Neill, R. E., & Starosta, K. (2005). Gathering functional assessment information. In L. M. Bambara & L. Kern (Eds.), *Individualized supports for students with problem behaviors* (pp. 129–164). New York: Guilford Press.

Lavigne, J. V., Arend, R., Rosenbaum, D., Binns, H., Christoffel, K. K., Kaufer, K., et al. (1998). Psychiatric disorders with onset in the preschool years: I. Stability of diagnoses. *Journal of the American Academy of Child and Adolescent Psychiatry, 37*(12), 1246–1254.

Loeber, R., & Dishion, T. (1983). Early predictors of male delinquency: A review. *Psychological Bulletin, 94*, 68–99.

Lucyshyn, J. M., Horner, R. H., Dunlap, G., Albin, R. W., & Ben, K. R. (2002). Positive behavior support with families. In J. M. Lucyshyn, G. Dunlap, & R. W. Albin (Eds.), *Families and positive behavior support: Addressing problem behavior in family contexts* (pp. 3–44). Baltimore: Brookes.

Lucyshyn, J. M., Kayser, A. T., Irvin, L. K., & Blumberg, E. R. (2002). Functional assessment and positive behavior support at home with families: Designing effective and contextually appropriate behavior support plans. In J. M. Lucyshyn, G. Dunlap, & R. W. Albin (Eds.), *Families and positive behavior support: Addressing problem behavior in family contexts* (pp. 97–132). Baltimore: Brookes.

McCormick, K. M., Jolivette, K., & Ridgley, R. (2003). Choice making as an intervention strategy for young children. *Young Exceptional Children, 6*(2), 3-10.

Mirenda, P., MacGregor, T., Kelly-Keough, S. (2002). Teaching communication skills or behavioral support in the context of family life. In J. M. Lucyshyn, G. Dunlap, & R. W.

Albin (Eds.), *Families and positive behavior support: Addressing problem behavior in family contexts* (pp. 185–208). Baltimore: Brookes.

Moffitt, T. E., Caspi, A., Dickson, N., Silva, P., & Stanton, W. (1996). Childhood-onset versus adolescent-onset antisocial conduct problems in males: Natural history from ages 3 to 18 years. *Development and Psychopathology, 8,* 399–424.

Moreland, A. D., & Dumas, J. E. (2008). Categorical and dimensional approaches to the measurement of disruptive behavior in the preschool years: A meta-analysis. *Clinical Psychology Review, 28,* 1059–1070.

Nielsen, S. L., Olive, M. L., Donovan, A., & McEvoy, M. (1998). Challenging behaviors in your classroom? Don't react—teach instead! *Young Exceptional Children, 2*(1), 2–10.

O'Neill, R. E., Horner, R. H., Albin, R. W., Storey, K., Sprague, J. R., & Newton, J. S. (1997). *Functional assessment of problem behavior: A practical assessment guide.* Pacific Grove, CA: Brooks/Cole.

O'Neill, R. E., Vaughn, B. J., & Dunlap, G. (1998). Comprehensive behavioral support: Assessment issues and strategies. In A. M. Wetherby, S. F. Warren, & J. Reichle (Eds.), *Transitions in prelinguistic communication* (pp. 313–341). Baltimore: Brookes.

Powell, D., Dunlap, G., & Fox, L. (2006). Prevention and intervention for the challenging behaviors of toddlers and preschoolers. *Infants and Young Children, 19*(1), 25–35.

Richman, N., Stevenson, J., & Graham, P. J. (1982). *Preschool to school: A behavioral study.* London: Academic Press.

Shaw, D. S., Gilliom, M., & Giovannelli, J. (2000). Aggressive behavior disorders. In C. H. Zeanah (Ed.), *Handbook of infant mental health* (2nd ed., pp. 397–411). New York: Guilford Press.

Turnbull, A. P., & Ruef, M. (1996). Family perspectives on problem behavior. *Mental Retardation, 34,* 280–293.

Turnbull, A. P., & Ruef, M. (1997). Family perspectives on inclusive lifestyle issues for people with problem behavior. *Exceptional Children, 63,* 211–227.

United States Department of Education. (2001). To assure the free appropriate public education of all children with disabilities. Individuals with Disabilities Act, Section 618. Twenty-third Annual Report to Congress on the Implementation of the Individuals with Disabilities Education Act.

United States Department of Education. (2002). To assure the free appropriate public education of all children with disabilities. Individuals with Disabilities Act, Section 618. Twenty-fourth Annual Report to Congress on the Implementation of the Individuals with Disabilities Education Act.

United States General Accounting Office. (2001). *Student discipline: Individuals with disabilities in education act* (GAO Report No. GAO-01-210). Washington, DC: Author.

Worcester, J. A., Nesman, T. M., Mendez, L. M. R., & Keller, H. R. (2008). Giving voice to parents of young children with challenging behaviors. *Exceptional Children, 74,* 509–525.

Home-Visiting Checklist:
Addressing Challenging Behavior

Home Visitor: _____ Date: _____

Observer: _____

Did the home visitor . . .	✓ ✗ ? NA	Notes
Understanding family concerns		
1. Initiate the conversation about challenging behavior by expressing concern about the child's ability to be engaged, communicate needs, self-regulate, etc.?		
2. Receive information from the family about challenging behavior without judgment or alarm?		
3. Allow the family to express their feelings about or reactions to the problem behavior without judgment or dismissal?		
4. Ask the family to identify the behaviors that they consider problematic?		
5. Validate family concerns and then offer to assist the family in developing strategies?		
6. Ask the family to describe the strategies or approaches they have used to resolve behavior problems and how well they have worked?		
7. Provide the family, when discussing their efforts to provide guidance to the child, with reassurance about parenting strengths?		
8. Ask the family to identify the routines or activities that are difficult for the child or the behaviors that cause the greatest concern?		
9. Provide information on problem behavior that is developmentally expected paired with an explanation of why the behavior can occur at that age?		

(cont.)

✓ = Done at a satisfactory level; ✗ = not done; ? = perhaps done or done but perhaps not at a satisfactory level; NA = not applicable.

Did the home visitor . . .	✓ ✗ ? NA	Notes
10. Provide the family with information on how to guide children when developmentally expected problem behavior is occurring?		
Providing information on positive parenting techniques		
11. Acknowledge family frustration with behavior by offering reflections on what you see (e.g., "It seems like Tanya really pushes your buttons when she throws her toys")?		
12. Provide the family with suggestions on how to handle stress about problem behavior that can lead to anger or inappropriate actions?		
13. Ask the family about their goals for parenting strategies for guiding behavior?		
14. Provide family with ideas about fostering engagement, communicating expectations, and developing routines that will promote the child's appropriate behavior?		
15. Provide the family with ideas about how to respond to problem behavior in a manner that is positive, firm, and does not provide a pay-off for problem behavior?		
16. Match recommended strategies with family needs and competing demands?		
17. Inquire about the behavioral progress of the child by asking open-ended questions about the routine or activity (e.g., "What are bedtimes like?")?		
18. Express confidence in the family's ability to implement new approaches to guiding behavior and reflect that change can take time?		
Developing support strategies for challenging behavior		
19. To gain an understanding of the family's expectations and desires, ask the family to identify what they would like a routine or activity to look like?		
20. Describe challenging behavior as serving a purpose for children and describe the need to do the "detective work" to determine why problem behavior is occurring?		
21. Ask the family to identify when the challenging behavior is most likely to occur, who it is most likely to occur with, and what interactions seem to trigger the behavior?		

(cont.)

Did the home visitor . . .	✓ ✗ ? NA	Notes
22. Engage the family in a conversation about what the purpose of challenging behavior might be and offer ideas?		
23. When providing information on support strategies, provide the family with information on why the child is engaging in challenging behavior (i.e., function)?		
24. Provide the family with concrete strategies for preventing challenging behavior and teaching replacement skills?		
25. Offer strategies that will be easy for family members to implement within everyday routines?		
26. Offer a simple written and verbal description of the use of a formal process for developing a behavior support plan if a plan will be needed?		
27. Develop written plans, charts, or visuals that will help the family remember strategies that they choose to implement?		
28. Offer to coach the family member through a problem behavior episode when it occurs during the visit?		
29. Warn the family that initial attempts to change behavior might be difficult for them to implement and that the child's behavior can get worse before it gets better?		
30. Encourage the family to implement the plan consistently?		
31. Provide encouragement to the family member after he or she has intervened with a problem behavior?		
32. When observing the implementation of the behavior support strategies, provide encouragement to the family?		
33. Ask the family to use simple outcome measures (e.g., rating scales or behavior charts) that document change in child-appropriate behaviors and reflect family goals?		
34. Review progress of the child and family efforts to implement the plan?		
35. Celebrate success with the family?		

Index

Page numbers in italics indicate tables or figures.

Accountability outcomes, 204
Activity settings
    in Contextually Mediated Practices, 64–67
    defined, 176
Advocacy services, informing families of, 107–108
Assessments, coordinating performance of, 96, 98–99
Audiologists, *104*

Backward-mapping, 204–206
Behavior expectations, 245, *246*

Caregiver benefits, 78
Caregiver responsiveness, 76–77
Caregiver Responsive Teaching Checklist, 76, *91*
Challenging behaviors
    addressing discipline techniques, 242–244
    assumptions regarding, 240
    developing a behavior support plan, 249–253
    dos and don'ts in talking to families about, *243*
    effect on the family, 238–239
    home visiting checklist, 257–259
    overview, 237–238
    responding to effectively, 247–249
    support framework, 239–240
    understanding family concerns about, 240–242
Change, diversity in views about, 160
Change question, 32
Childhood intervention, 62
Child-instruction strategies, 220–221
Child interests, identifying, 73–74

Child Interests Checklist, 73, 88
Child learning
    contextualized and decontextualized, 65
    increasing opportunities, 69
    interest-based, 67–69
    parent-mediated, 69–70
    peripheral, 67
Child rearing, 159
Children
    diversity in views about, 159
    in poverty, 150
CMP. *See* Contextually Mediated Practices
Coaching
    action/practice and, 180
    case example, 190–193
    challenges to the field of, 193–196
    checklist, 201–202
    concept of, 177–178
    cost issues, 193
    definitions of, 177–179
    determining the frequency, intensity and duration
        of visits, 189–190
    effective teaming characteristics, 181–183
    feedback and, 180–181
    goal of, 178
    identifyling primary coaches, 187–190
    implementation conditions, 183–184
    implementation steps, 184–190
    joint planning and, 179
    observation and, 179–180

Coaching *(cont.)*
    operational definition, 176
    payment issues, 193–194
    program leadership and, 194
    reflection and, 180
    role of, 178
Collaborative child care consultation, 206–207
Communication
    culturally competent service delivery and, 156–
        158
    diversity in styles, 156–158
    informal, 128–130
    See also Consultations; Talking to families
Community activities, identifying, 74
Competence
    child, 70, 78
    parent, 71, 78
    See also Cross-cultural competence
Confidence
    child, 71, 78
    parent, 71, 78
Consequences, logical, 249
Consultations
    CMP implementation and practice, 71–79
    coaching families, 177–181 (*see also* Coaching)
    collaborative child care consultation, 206–207
    in culturally competent service delivery, 161–168
    with families about supports, 12–13
    with families of children with challenging
        behavior, 240–244
    in home visiting (*see* Support-based home visiting)
    routines-based interview, 30–36
    in service coordination (*see* Service coordination)
    talking to families (*see* Talking to families)
    transdisciplinary team in the primary provider
        model, 104–105
    See also Communication
Context specific learning, 61
Contextualized learning, 65
Contextually Mediated Practices (CMP)
    checklists, 72–73, 99–92
    child interests, 67–69
    evaluation, 77–78
    everyday activity settings, 64–67
    factors limiting the wide use of, 80–81
    feedback, 78–79
    guiding principles, 62–63
    implementation, 75–77
    likelihood of use by parents and caregivers, 79–80
    origin, 61
    outcomes and benefits, 70–71
    overview, 63–64
    parent-mediated child learning, 69–70
    phases of, 71–72
    planning, 73–75
Cross-cultural competence
    definitions, 154
    developing, 154–155
Cultural continua, 152–153
Cultural diversity, 151–153

Culturally competent service delivery
    beliefs about disability or risk conditions and,
        159–160
    beliefs about family roles and, 158
    checklists, 172–174
    communication styles and, 156–158
    data gathering and assessment, 162–163, *164–165*
    example situations, 168–169
    home-based services, 167–168
    initial contact, 162
    intervention plan development, 163, 166
    intervention plan implementation, 166–167
    monitoring and evaluation, 167
    significance of, 161–162
    and views about change and interventions, 160–
        161
    and views about children and child rearing, 159

Decontextualized learning, 65
Diagnostic assessments, 98
Disability, diversity in beliefs about, 159–160
Discipline, 242–244
Diversity
    associations among family characteristics and, 153
    in beliefs about disability or risk conditions,
        159–160
    in beliefs about family roles, 158
    building relationships with families, 156–161
    cultural components, 151–153
    defining, 147–148
    in family structure and family members, 148–149
    in sociocultural factors, 150–151
    in styles of communication, 156–158
    in views about change and interventions, 160–161
    in views about children and child rearing, 159

Early childhood special education teachers, *104*
Early intervention programs, funding challenges,
        193
Ecology, 9–10
Ecomaps
    checklist, 25–26
    clarifying early interventions with, 21–22
    constructing, 16–19
    determining goals for the future with, 20–21
    determining the need for additional supports and,
        19–20
    evaluating outcomes and measuring change with,
        21
    example, *15*
    intervention planning and, 19
    overview, 13–14
    preparation for developing, 15
    significance of, 22
    ways to facilitate, 14
Eligibility assessments, 98
Emotional support, 11
Engagement, 30, 218–219
"Errorless learning," 221
Ethics, 167

Evaluations, coordinating performance of, 96, 98–99
Everyday activity participation, 77–78
Everyday activity settings, 64–67
Everyday community learning, *66*
Everyday Community Learning Activity Checklist, 74, 89

FACINATE model, 206–207, 209
Families
    diversity in, 148–149
    traditional definition, 149
    U.S. statistics on, 149
Family-level outcomes, 40–41, 102–103
Family-professional partnerships, 127–128
Family roles, diversity in beliefs about, 158
Family structure, 148–149
Family support
    categories, 10–12
    conversations with families about, 12–13
    sources, *17*
Feedback, performance, 223–224
First responders, 162
Follow-up questions, 35
Formal support, 12
Functional assessments, 99
Functional child domains
    engagement, 218–219
    independence, 219
    social relationships, 219
Functional child outcomes, 38–40
Functional needs assessment, 27–29
Future ecomaps, 20–21

Health care, diversity in views about, 160–161
Health providers
    coordinating services with, 108–109
    See also Medical providers
High-context cultures, 156
Home-based services
    culturally competent, 167–168
    See also Home visiting
Home–school communication, 130
Home visiting
    backward-mapping approach, 204–206
    in early intervention, 203–207
    FACINATE context, 206–207
    families who don't follow through with
        interventions and, 224
    families who have been coerced into services and, 224–225
    families who want more than can be offered and, 225–226
    families with multiple needs and, 225
    guidelines for visitors, *164–165*
    key principles, 208–209
    misplaced clinic-based approach, 207–208
    recommendations for success in, 226
    three-tiered approach, 221–223
    Vanderbilt Home Visit Script, 212–218
    See also Support-based home visiting

IEP. *See* Individualized education program
IFSP. *See* Individualized family service plan
IFSP meeting, 100, 101–103
IFSP outcomes
    selection issues, 195–196
    team-based development, 186–187
    writing, 102–103
IFSP teams
    agendas and, 101
    keeping printed minutes, 101
    mission statements, 101
    preparing for meetings, 101–102
Ignoring, planned, 247–248
Incidental teaching, 220–221
Increasing Everyday Child Learning Opportunities
        Checklist, 75–76, 90
Independence, 219
Individualized education program (IEP)
    conversations with families about supports and,
        12–13
    functional needs assessment and, 27–29
Individualized family service plan (IFSP)
    accountability, 93
    conversations with families about supports and,
        12–13
    conversion from shorthand to IFSP wording, *40*
    development, review, and evaluation, 99–103
    family-level outcomes and the RBI, 40–41
    functional needs assessment and, 27–29
    issues in developing, 195–196
    outcomes, 102–103
    purpose, 93
    strategy planning and, 34
Individuals with Disabilities Education Act (IDEA)
        Part C programs, 93
    CMP-type interventions and, 80
    family outcomes, 102
Informal support, 12
Informational support, 11–12
Integrated assessments, 99
Interest-based learning, 67–69, 75, 177
Intervention plans/planning
    in culturally competent service delivery, 163,
        166–167
    ecomaps and, 19
Interventions
    distinguished from services, 208
    diversity in views about, 160–161

Languages, statistics on, 152
Lead questions, 213–215
Learning environments, natural, 61
Logical consequences, 249
Logic model of service coordination, 95–96, *97*,
        110
Low-context cultures, 156

Material support, 11
Mediation, components, 70
Medical home, 108

Medical providers
    coordinating services with, 108–109
    in early intervention, *104*
Misplaced clinic-based approach, 207–208
Model-and-pray approach, 216
Modeling, eight steps of, 216–217
Moral outcomes, 204–205
Multidisciplinary teams, 98–99

Natural learning environment practices, 176–177
Natural learning environments, 61, 190
Nutritionists, *104*

Occupational therapists, *104*

Parenting techniques, positive, 244–247
Parent-mediated child learning, 69–70
Parent-Mediated Child Learning Evaluation
    Checklist, 77, 92
Parent-professional partnerships
    disagreements and, 136–137
    interpersonal factors and, 127–128
Parents
    soliciting ideas and opinions from, 133–134
    teaching parents to teach their children, 219–224
Participation, 70, 218
People networks, 16–17
Performance feedback, 223–224
Peripheral learning, 67
Personal interests, 67
Physical therapists, *104*
Planned ignoring, 247–248
Positive behavior support
    behavior hypothesis, 250–251
    coaching and modeling, 252
    functional assessment, 250
    monitoring implementation and outcomes, 252–
        253
    overview, 249–250
    support plan development, 251–252
Positive parenting techniques
    praise, 244–245
    prevention strategies, 246–247
    teaching behavior expectations, 245, *246*
Poverty, 150
Praise, 244–245
Preservice educators, 195
Primary language, 152
Primary service provider, 103–106, 175
Psychologists, *104*

Race, 151
RBI. *See* Routine-Based Interview
RBI Implementation Checklist, 44–47
RBI Report Form, 36–37, 48–50
RBI-SAFER Combo, 51–59
Redirection, 248–249
Reinforcement, 221
Replacement skills, 251
Risk conditions, 159–160

Role release, 106
Roundtables, 167
Routine-Based Interview (RBI), 214
    defined, 27, 29
    documenting results, 36–41
    examples of informal outcomes, 37–38
    family interview, 30–32
    implementation challenges and solutions, 41
    key statements and questions, 35–36
    keys to a successful interview, 34–35
    preparation for, 29
    significance of, 41–42
    teacher interviews, 32–34
    writing a family-level outcome from, 40–41
    writing a functional child outcome from, 38–40
Routines, 29

Self-awareness, 154–155
Service, distinguished from intervention, 208
Service coordination
    assisting families in choosing service providers,
        103–106
    checklists, 112–126
    coordinating with medical and health providers,
        108–109
    defined, 94
    ecological framework, 95
    evaluation, 110
    informing families of advocacy services, 107–108
    logic model, 95–96, *97*, 110
    multidisciplinary teams, 98–99
    outcomes, *95*
    performing evaluations and assessments, 96, 98–
        99
    research foundation for, 94–96
    service delivery and, 106–107
    transition plans and, 109
Service Coordination, Research and Training Center
    on, 94–96
Service coordinators, responsibilities, 93–94, 99–100
Service providers
    assisting families in choosing, 103–106
    differences between educational level of providers
        and families, 150
Situated learning, 61
Situational interests, 67
Social networks, 16–17
Social relationships, 30–31, 219
Social workers, *104*
Speech-language pathologists, *104*
Spirit Catches You and You Fall Down, The (Fadiman),
    161
Strategy planning
    IFSPs and, 34
    Routine-Based Interviews and, 34
Support
    emotional, 210–211
    informational, 211–212
    material, 211
    See also Family support

Support-based home visiting
    assumptions, 209–210
    eight steps of modeling, 216–217
    hands-on contact with children, 215–217
    implications for specialists' roles, 217–218
    providing emotional support, 210–211
    providing informational support, 211–212
    providing material support, 211
    teaching parents to teach their children, 219–224
    transdisciplinary service delivery, 217
    Vanderbilt Home Visit Script, 212–218, 233–236
    See also Home visiting

"Tag-along" activities, 67
Talking to families
    acknowledge and respond to feelings, 140–142
    acknowledge child and family strengths, 130–132
    checklist, 144–146
    demonstrate caring for the whole family, 137–140
    informal exchange, 128–130
    seek understanding, 134–137
    solicit parents' opinions and ideas, 133–134
Teacher interviews, 32–34

Team leaders, 185
Team meetings, 185
Teams
    developing participation-based IFSP outcomes, 186–187
    effective characteristics, 181–183
    identifying, 184–185
    information gathering and, 186
    significance of, 181
    widespread acceptance of, 175
    See also Primary-coach approach to teaming
Team size, 182–183
Team tasks, 182
Three-tiered approach, to home visits, 221–223
Time delay, 221
Transdisciplinary service delivery, 217
Transdisciplinary teams, 104–105
Transition plans, 109
Transitions, 109

Vanderbilt Home Visit Script, 212–218, 233–236

When-then statements, 248
Worry question, 31